Palgrave Studies in Cyberpsychology

Series Editor

Jens Binder, Nottingham Trent University, Nottingham, UK

Palgrave Studies in Cyberpsychology aims to foster and to chart the scope of research driven by a psychological understanding of the effects of the 'new technology' that is shaping our world after the digital revolution. The series takes an inclusive approach and considers all aspects of human behaviours and experiential states in relation to digital technologies, to the Internet, and to virtual environments. As such, Cyberpsychology reaches out to several neighbouring disciplines, from Human-Computer Interaction to Media and Communication Studies. A core question underpinning the series concerns the actual psychological novelty of new technology. To what extent do we need to expand conventional theories and models to account for cyberpsychological phenomena? At which points is the ubiquitous digitisation of our everyday lives shifting the focus of research questions and research needs? Where do we see implications for our psychological functioning that are likely to outlast shortlived fashions in technology use?

Elizabeth Sillence · Alison Osborne

Digital Health Technologies and the Menopause

palgrave
macmillan

Elizabeth Sillence
Psychology Department
Northumbria University
Newcastle upon Tyne, UK

Alison Osborne
Psychology Department
Northumbria University
Newcastle upon Tyne, UK

ISSN 2946-2754 ISSN 2946-2762 (electronic)
Palgrave Studies in Cyberpsychology
ISBN 978-3-032-25908-0 ISBN 978-3-032-25909-7 (eBook)
https://doi.org/10.1007/978-3-032-25909-7

The authors declare that financial support was received for the research, authorship, and publication of this book. This work was funded by the EPSRC Centre for Digital Citizens (grant number EP/T022582/1).

This Palgrave Macmillan imprint is published by the registered company Springer Nature Switzerland AG
The registered company address is: Gewerbestrasse 11, 6330 Cham, Switzerland

Acknowledgements We would like to thank the following people for their contributions to our ongoing work in this space. Kerry Lakey, Emma Kemp, Richard Brown, Niamh Harvey, Caroline Claisse, Abi Durrant, and Shahla Rushworth and all the women who gave their time to talk to us about their experiences.

Competing Interests The authors have no competing interests to declare that are relevant to the content of this manuscript.

Contents

List of Tables

1

Introduction

Abstract Menopause is a topic that is receiving increased attention across the media, politics, medicine, and retail. Despite this attention, many women still report feeling underprepared and lack sufficient knowledge to help them navigate menopause. This book sets out to examine the role of digital health technologies as a source of information and support for women. We begin in this chapter by introducing menopause, outlining traditional sources of menopause information and then highlighting the increasing use of digital health technologies in menopause information and support. The aim here is to set the scene for discussing the evolving role of digital health technologies in this space in light of current narratives in menopause. Having set the scene for the rest of the book, the chapter closes by briefly introducing the upcoming chapters.

Keywords Menopause · Digital health technologies · Health information seeking · Media representation · Menopausal narratives

E. Sillence and A. Osborne, *Digital Health Technologies and the Menopause*, Palgrave Studies in Cyberpsychology, https://doi.org/10.1007/978-3-032-25909-7_1

1.1 Introduction

Menopause, characterised by the point in time where a woman's menstrual periods have stopped for 12 consecutive months (World Health Organization, 2024), usually occurs in a woman's late forties or early fifties in Western Cultures, with around 1 in 100 women experiencing menopause prior to the age of 40 years (Hardy et al., 2018). The age at which women experience menopause can be highly variable, and menopause can be induced as a result of surgery, serious illness, or medication (Hoga et al., 2015; Hunter et al., 2012). Menopause is heterogeneous, with some women experiencing few or no symptoms whereas for others it impacts the normal functioning and quality of life (Ayers & Hunter, 2013; Duffy et al., 2011; Marnocha et al., 2011; O'Reilly et al., 2023). Symptoms of menopause include hot flushes, anxiety, fatigue, brain fog, weight gain, and migraines (Hunter, 2019; Marlatt et al., 2018) and can begin several years prior to menopause, during a period known as perimenopause so that in an ageing population, women spend one third of their lives perimenopausal, menopausal, or postmenopausal (Gold, 2011). Hormone Replacement Therapy (HRT) is the main medicine treatment for menopause and perimenopause symptoms. Talking therapies such as Cognitive Behavioural Therapy (CBT) and lifestyle interventions can also help with physical symptoms such as hot flushes and with low mood and anxiety. Non-hormonal medicines include Selective Serotonin Reuptake Inhibitors (SSRIs,) and there are a number of alternative therapies including dietary supplements or herbal remedies, acupuncture, and meditation (NHS, 2025).

Given the heterogeneity of experiences around symptoms, it is not surprising that women report differing perspectives and experiences with respect to menopause. Women can feel positive towards menopause, accepting of it, or express negative or fearful emotions (Tariq et al., 2023). A study of UK mothers by de Salis et al. (2018) identified three interdependent narratives around menopause: (1) normality—menopause as a normal, biological process distinct from self, identity, and social transitions; (2) distress—menopause as a struggle provoking and expressing distress, a time of identity loss and social upheaval; (3) transformation—menopause as a time of liberation and transformation.

Women might shift between narratives, either experiencing them simultaneously or successively, although often one dominates. A systematic review of women's menopausal experiences in the UK (Anto et al., 2025) showed that women's experiences are shaped by the biopsychosocial dimensions of menopause, including the impact on their professional and personal relationships, their understanding of menopause, often shaped by the symptoms experienced as well as that of their mother, and their strategies to menopause management including interactions with Healthcare Professionals (HCPs).

Whilst the incidence and severity of menopausal symptoms are related to a number of individual factors, including health status, socio-cultural characteristics are also important. Attitudes towards menopause affect experience of specific symptoms, and women going into perimenopause with more negative expectations are more likely to experience difficult symptoms (Ayers et al., 2010). Likewise, menopause is often experienced negatively in cultures where fertility is particularly valued (Khademi & Cooke, 2003). A review of sex and sexual relationships in menopause noted both positive and negative meanings for women across different countries, including no fear of pregnancy or need for contraception, but associations with an ageing body, loss of femininity, and lack of interest in sex (Bulut et al., 2025). Menopause is considered a negative concept in China, with women being subject to verbal and physical abuse and menopause being deemed almost equivalent to craziness or mental illness (Li et al., 2023), although interestingly, listening to podcasts improved women's own perceptions and emotional experiences of menopause (Guo & Li, 2024).

1.1.1 Menopause as a 'Hot Topic'

Commentators and academics agree that menopause is currently a hot topic in the UK (Orgad & Rottenberg, 2024). Recent television programmes presented by Davina McCall (Channel 4, 2021) have been credited with removing the historical stigma around menopause and have even led to the so-called 'Davina effect', a rush on HRT requests which led to national shortages (Jermyn, 2025). This so-called menopause movement has seen menopause move from a topic barely mentioned to one that is visible across traditional media and social media (Hunter et al., 2023), politics, medicine, and retail. This cultural shift is captured in Jermyn's (2023) term 'the menopausal turn'.

This more open approach to menopause is to be welcomed but has brought with it accusations of 'menowashing' (Daily Mail, 2024) and intense commercialisation (Panay et al., 2024; Pleace, 2024) as retailers, celebrities, and other menopause 'experts' launch 'menopause friendly' products and services. It has also reignited a debate about the way in which the menopause is portrayed. One narrative presents menopause in a highly medicalised manner, essentially a hormone deficiency that is treatable (for most women). Another portrays menopause as a normal life transition, one that may or may not need medical support, and other narratives advocate for menopause as a time of potential transformation free from the constraints of menstrual cycles.

1.1.2 Sources of Menopause Information

Information about menopause can be conflicting, both around experiences and symptomology. Women often indicate poor knowledge and awareness of the menopause transition and its treatments (Bakouei et al., 2013; Duffy et al., 2011; Herbert et al., 2020; Marnocha et al., 2011; Tariq et al., 2023). This can affect women's perceptions of their experience (Buchanan et al., 2002) and the likelihood that they will seek or receive the medical assistance they require (Marnocha et al., 2011). Feelings of embarrassment, perceived adverse reactions from others, and cultural taboos also act as barriers to support (Bidmon & Terlutter, 2015; Timmermans, 2020).

Previously, women have relied on family and friends for information and support about menopause. For example, Dillaway (2007, p. 91) found that "women used their knowledge of mothers' experiences as a benchmark for understanding, defining, and manoeuvring this reproductive transition". Opportunities for discussion have increased with a generational shift in openness towards talking about reproductive health milestones (Field-Springer et al., 2018). Hayfield et al. (2024) explored the role of friends, family, and relationships on women's experiences of menopause, noting that women discussed a sense of solidarity based on shared, embodied experiences, something the authors termed the 'menopause sisterhood'.

Most women start to seek information about menopause once symptoms start to appear (Harper et al., 2022) and have sought that information from friends, HCPs, and online resources. The internet is now the go-to place for health information, with individuals searching on websites and social media before consulting healthcare professionals (Jacobs et al., 2017). The COVID-19 pandemic has accelerated the provision of digital resources for menopause, and it is clear that women are using websites, social media (Harper et al., 2022), and mobile health apps (Sillence et al., 2023) for menopause information and support. A recent review (Osborne & Sillence, 2025) suggested women find these digital resources accessible, convenient, and easy to use and helped women to normalise, validate, and legitimise their own menopause experience as well as to understand their symptoms.

And so, the focus of this book is on the role of digital health technologies (DHTs) for menopause information and support. Digital health technologies take many different forms (DTx, 2023) and, for menopause, can include digital bracelets and digital clothing as well as mobile apps and websites (Lopez Burst et al., 2024). The focus of this book is on technologies to support digital health communication rather than on products designed to, for example, alleviate hot flushes (for an interesting discussion on these kinds of products, see Zhang et al., 2025 and Lopez Burst et al., 2024, and for ideas about the future design of products for menopause, see work from KTH in Sweden, e.g. Ciolfi Felice et al., 2021). In the context of the 'menopausal turn', we ask what is the role of DHTs in menopause information and support? What do different DHTs offer women, how well do they cover the topics women want to know about, and how well do they represent the women seeking information? Each chapter focuses on a different DHT to look for similarities and differences in how women experience these digital resources and assess their value in supporting women through menopause. Throughout this book, we use the terms woman and women, but we recognise that menopause affects trans and gender diverse people. We also acknowledge that our studies are situated within a UK context and reflect upon this point in the final chapter.

The rest of the book is organised as follows: In Chapter 2, we examine online information for menopause. We look at search results to get a flavour of the websites that individuals may encounter and discuss the literature on evaluating online health information. We then focus on menopause information online and present findings from one of our recent studies that captures the search process women go through when looking online, their evaluation strategies, and the type of websites and content they discover.

In Chapter 3, we introduce mobile health (mHealth) and the potential role of menopause smartphone apps in health communication. Starting with women's health more broadly, we then focus on the landscape of menopause apps including features, functionality, and healthcare professional input. Drawing on examples from our own research, looking at women's experiences of using menopause apps, we demonstrate how women are using the different features of the apps to support their menopause journeys.

In Chapter 4, we provide an overview of the menopause podcast landscape, noting key podcast series and topics. We present some findings from our recent work exploring women's preferences and experiences engaging with menopause information via podcasts. We detail how women find and select relevant podcasts, how they engage with the format, and how they evaluate the information they encounter. We reflect on the format itself and discuss how the distinct features of different resources may present specific opportunities to users.

In Chapter 5, we take a closer look at social media and menopause resources. We explore the expanding role of celebrities and influencers using social media to discuss menopause. We critique the notion of 'expertise' and empowerment in this context before considering how women respond to social media messaging. We detail a recent study on social media narratives and reflect on the way in which menopause continues to be repositioned across the media.

In Chapter 6, the focus switches to online peer support for menopause. Here, we introduce online peer support in its different forms and detail some examples of menopause peer support. We examine the literature around the benefits of engaging with online peer support and present some data on peer support engagement in the context of menopause.

Finally, in Chapter 7, we bring together our learning to evaluate how the different digital health technologies examined in the book play a role in menopause information and support and how they contribute to the current debates around medicalisation, empowerment, and representation. We reflect on the current gaps in the literature and identify potential limitations with the current research base. The chapter concludes by highlighting ongoing areas of research and suggesting practical and novel ways of integrating DHTs into in-person support.

References

Anto, A., Basu, A., Selim, R., & Eisingerich, A. B. (2025). Women's menopausal experiences in the UK: A systemic literature review of qualitative studies. *Health Expectations, 28(1), Article e70167.*

Ayers, B., Forshaw, M., & Hunter, M. S. (2010). The impact of attitudes towards the menopause on women's symptom experience: A systematic review. *Maturitas, 65*(1), 28–36.

Ayers, B. A., & Hunter, M. S. (2013). Health-related quality of life of women with menopausal hot flushes and night sweats. *Climacteric, 16*(2), 235–239.

Bakouei, F., Basirat, Z., Salmalian, H., Omidvar, S., & Bakouei, S. (2013). Assessment of women's awareness level about symptoms and complications of menopause and methods to their prevention. Journal of local and Global Health Science, 2013(1), Article 6.

Bidmon, S., & Terlutter, R. (2015). Gender differences in searching for health information on the internet and the virtual patient-physician relationship in Germany: Exploratory results on how men and women differ and why. Journal of Medical Internet Research, 17(6), Article e156.

Buchanan, M. C., Morris Villagran, M., & Ragan, S. L. (2002). Women, menopause, and (Ms.) information: Communication about the climacteric. *Health Communication, 14*(1), 99–119.

Bulut, H., Hinchliff, S., Ali, P., & Piercy, H. (2025). Women's experiences of intimate and sexual relationships during menopause: A qualitative synthesis. *Journal of Clinical Nursing, 34*(5), 1543–1554.

Channel l4. (2021). *Davina McCall: Sex, myths and the menopause*. https://www.channel4.com/programmes/davina-mccall-sex-myths-and-the-menopause

Ciolfi Felice, M., Søndergaard, M. L. J., & Balaam, M. (2021, May). Resisting the medicalisation of menopause: Reclaiming the body through design. Proceedings of the 2021 CHI conference on human factors in computing systems (pp. 1–16).

de Salis, I., Owen-Smith, A., Donovan, J. L., & Lawlor, D. A. (2018). Experiencing menopause in the UK: The interrelated narratives of normality, distress, and transformation. *Journal of Women & Aging, 30*(6), 520–540.

Dillaway, H. E. (2007). "am I similar to my mother?" how women make sense of menopause using family background. *Women & Health, 46*(1), 79–97.

DTx Alliance. (2023). Guidance to industry: Classification of digital health technologies, https://dtxalliance.org/wp-content/uploads/ 2023/06/Guidance-to-Industry-Classification-of-Digital-Health-Technologies-2023Jun05.pdf.

Duffy, O., Iversen, L., & Hannaford, P. C. (2011). The menopause 'it's somewhere between a taboo and a joke. *A focus group study. Climacteric, 14*(4), 497–505.

Field-Springer, K., Randall-Griffiths, D., & Reece, C. (2018). From menarche to menopause: Understanding multigenerational reproductive health milestones. *Health Communication, 33*(6), 733–742.

Gold, E. B. (2011). The timing of the age at which natural menopause occurs. *Obstetrics and Gynecology Clinics of North America, 38*(3), 425–440.

Guo, W., & Li, N. (2024, October). The impact of podcast media on Chinese women's perception and attitudes towards menopause in the digital era. In *19th world congress on menopause, international menopause society*.

Hardy, C., Thorne, E., Griffiths, A., & Hunter, M. (2018). Tackling the taboo: Talking menopause-related problems at work. *International Journal of Workplace Health Management, 12*(1), 28–38.

Harper, J. C., Phillips, S., Biswakarma, R., Yasmin, E., Saridogan, E., Radhakrishnan, S., & Talaulikar, V. (2022). An online survey of perimenopausal women to determine their attitudes and knowledge of the menopause. *Women's Health, 18*, Article 17455057221106890.

Hayfield, N., Moore, H., & Terry, G. (2024). "friends? Supported. Partner? Not so much...": Women's experiences of friendships, family, and relationships during perimenopause and menopause. *Feminism & Psychology, 34*(3), 443–463.

Herbert, D., Bell, R. J., Young, K., Brown, H., Coles, J. Y., & Davis, S. R. (2020). Australian women's understanding of menopause and its consequences: A qualitative study. *Climacteric, 23*(6), 622–628.

Hoga, L., Rodolpho, J., Gonçalves, B., & Quirino, B. (2015). Women's experience of menopause: A systematic review of qualitative evidence. *JBI Evidence Synthesis, 13*(8), 250–337.

Hunter, M. (2019). Menopause and midlife: Psychosocial perspectives and interventions. In *Routledge international handbook of women's sexual and reproductive health* (pp. 83–98). Routledge.

Hunter, M., Gentry-Maharaj, A., Ryan, A., Burnell, M., Lanceley, A., Fraser, L., Jacobs, I., & Menon, U. (2012). Prevalence, frequency and problem rating of hot flushes persist in older postmenopausal women: Impact of age, body mass index, hysterectomy, hormone therapy use, lifestyle and mood in a cross-sectional cohort study of 10,418 British women aged 54–65. *BJOG: An International Journal of Obstetrics & Gynaecology, 119*(1), 40–50.

Hunter, M. S., El-Haj, M., Thorne, E., Griffiths, A., & Hardy, C. (2023). # Menopause: Examining the frequency of communications about menopause on twitter between 2014 and 2022. *Maturitas, 177*, 107806. https://doi.org/10.1016/j.maturitas.2023.107806

Jacobs, W., Amuta, A. O., & Jeon, K. C. (2017). Health information seeking in the digital age: An analysis of health information seeking behavior among US adults. *Cogent. Social Sciences, 3*(1), Article 1302785.

Jermyn, D. (2023). 'Everything you need to embrace the change': *The 'menopausal turn' in contemporary UK culture. Journal of Aging Studies, 64*, Article 101114.

Jermyn, D. (2025). Whose menopause revolution? Investigating the UK'S 'Davina effect' and the contemporary menopause market. *European Journal of Cultural Studies, 28*(4), 1039–1057.

Khademi, S., & Cooke, M. S. (2003). Comparing the attitudes of urban and rural Iranian women toward menopause. *Maturitas, 46*(2), 113–121.

Li, Q., Gu, J., Huang, J., Zhao, P., & Luo, C. (2023). "they see me as mentally ill": The stigmatization experiences of Chinese menopausal women in the family. *BMC Women's Health, 23*(1), Article 185.

Lopez Burst, E., Ciolfi Felice, M., & O'Kane, A. A. (2024, May). Using and appropriating technology to support the menopause journey in the UK. *Proceedings of the CHI conference on human factors in computing systems* (pp. 1–14).

Daily Mail. (2024). 'An insult to women': Holland & Barrett accused of 'menowashing' with. £3.79 chocolate-covered 'menopause almond' bar that claims to ease hormonal changes.https://www.dailymail.co.uk/health/article-13456161/insult-women-Holland-Barrett-menowashing-chocolate-menopause-almond.html

Marlatt, K. L., Beyl, R. A., & Redman, L. M. (2018). A qualitative assessment of health behaviors and experiences during menopause: A cross-sectional, observational study. *Maturitas, 116*, 36–42.

Marnocha, S. K., Bergstrom, M., & Dempsey, L. F. (2011). The lived experience of perimenopause and menopause. *Contemporary Nurse, 37*(2), 229–240.

NHS. (2025). *Menopause.* https://www.nhs.uk/conditions/menopause/

O'Reilly, K., McDermid, F., McInnes, S., & Peters, K. (2023). An exploration of women's knowledge and experience of perimenopause and menopause: An integrative literature review. *Journal of Clinical Nursing, 32*(15–16), 4528–4540.

Orgad, S., & Rottenberg, C. (2024). The menopause moment: The rising visibility of 'the change' in UK news coverage. *European Journal of Cultural Studies, 27*(4), 519–539.

Osborne, A. K., & Sillence, E. (2025). Accessing information on menopause transition and the role of digital health technologies: A narrative review. *Women & Health*, 1–14.

Panay, N., Ang, S. B., Cheshire, R., Goldstein, S. R., Maki, P., Nappi, R. E., & International Menopause Society Board. (2024). Menopause and MHT in 2024: Addressing the key controversies—An international menopause society white paper. *South African General Practitioner, 5*(3), 119–134.

Pleace, K. (2024). Why celebrity menopause activism can hinder as well as help women. *The Conversation.* https://theconversation.com/why-celebrity-menopause-activism-can-hinder-as-well-as-help-women-225974

Sillence, E., Hardy, C., & Kemp, E. (2023). "this app just gets me": Assessing the quality, features and user reviews of menopause smartphone apps. *Journal of Consumer Health On The Internet, 27*(2), 156–172.

Tariq, B., Phillips, S., Biswakarma, R., Talaulikar, V., & Harper, J. C. (2023). Women's knowledge and attitudes to the menopause: A comparison of women over 40 who were in the perimenopause, post menopause and those not in the peri or post menopause. *BMC Women's Health, 23*(1), Article 460.

Timmermans, S. (2020). The engaged patient: The relevance of patient–physician communication for twenty-first-century health. *Journal of Health and Social Behavior, 61*(3), 259–273.

World Health Organization. (2024). *Menopause.* https://www.who.int/news-room/fact-sheets/detail/menopause

Zhang, W., Bao, H., Li, C., Zhai, Y., Liu, J., & Gong, J. (2025, April). Exploring wearable design for emotional health and well-being during menopause: Perspectives and design opportunities. *Proceedings of the extended abstracts of the CHI conference on human factors in computing systems* (pp. 1–9).

2
Online Information for Menopause

Abstract In this chapter, we paint a picture of the current landscape of online information around menopause. Many women report feeling underprepared for menopause, and health websites can therefore be a key digital information resource for women seeking information and support for their health (Lupton & Maslen, 2019). This chapter provides readers with an overview of the types of information, the sources, and providers of menopause information currently available. The chapter is organised as follows: (1) We introduce health websites as a valuable resource for women going through menopause and provide an overview of some of the current websites available. (2) In this section, we discuss how women make decisions about what online information and advice to trust. (3) We then present information on how women search for and evaluate menopause information online and explore how the content of the sites they encounter differs, drawing on data from a recent study we conducted. We conclude by reflecting on the website types and the topics covered and note changes in the online menopause information landscape over the last 20 years.

Keywords Online health information · Menopause websites · Search strategies · Source credibility · Trust evaluation

E. Sillence and A. Osborne, *Digital Health Technologies and the Menopause*, Palgrave Studies in Cyberpsychology, https://doi.org/10.1007/978-3-032-25909-7_2

2.1 Health Websites for Menopause

Whilst family and friends are the most common source of information on the menopause for under 40 s, approximately half of over 20 s report using websites for their menopause information (Munn et al., 2022). Other studies have indicated that around 60% of perimenopausal women have looked on health websites for menopause information (Harper et al., 2022), although far fewer have used official websites, e.g. professional society websites such as the British Menopause Society or their patient arm, Women's Health Concern (Tariq et al., 2023). Post menopausal women are also using health websites for menopause information (Tariq et al., 2023), collectively indicating that health websites are a well-used source of information for women during the menopause.

These surveys and others (Davies & Halliday, 2025) identify a number of 'official' and 'unofficial' websites that women report using in relation to menopause, but do not often provide details on the specific websites visited or the sites that are returned during an online search.

We conducted a Google search for 'menopause' and 'menopause and HRT' (11th March 2025, UK-based search), which returned the following information (see Table 2.1).

The 'Menopause' search returned the NHS website as the first result. The other search results returned on page one represented a range of countries, and organisations include charities, professional bodies, and non-UK healthcare providers. The Google search also indicated what 'people also ask' and what 'people also search for'. These queries and search terms reveal concerns around the timeline of menopause, identifying menopausal symptoms, and a few treatment-related questions.

'Menopause and HRT' returned a sponsored link to 'The menopause clinic', but also returned links to many of the same websites as the 'menopause search'. The 'people also ask' and what 'people also search for' queries were dominated by HRT, although natural menopause treatments were also included here.

Looking at the NHS website (https://www.nhs.uk/conditions/menopause/) in more detail, we see it is split into overview, symptoms, things you can do, treatment, and help and support. These

Table 2.1 Search results for Menopause and Menopause and HRT

	'Menopause'	'Menopause and HRT'
Search results	NHS website MayoClinic National Institute on ageing Cleveland Clinic WHO British menopause society The menopause charity Wikipedia	The menopause clinic NHS website Cleveland clinic Mayo clinic British menopause society The menopause society My menopause Centre Australasian menopause society NHSinform Scotland Wikipedia
People also ask	What are the 5 stages of menopause? How to reduce menopause symptoms? Will I feel better after menopause? Can you manage menopause without HRT?	What is the downside of HRT for menopause? What happens if you don't take HRT during menopause? What does HRT do for menopause? Which HRT is best for menopause?
People also search for	Menopause vitamins Signs of menopause at 40 Menopause symptoms, What are the 1st signs of menopause? What signals the end of menopause? Menopause age Menopause symptoms 47 How long does menopause last?	What are the signs you need hormone replacement therapy? Menopause without HRT Perimenopause HRT and periods Pros and cons of HRT Do I need HRT quiz? 7 natural menopause treatments that really work Benefits of HRT after 65 HRT medication names

sections cover the basics of the menopause journey, mental and physical symptoms, self-care strategies, HRT and non-hormonal treatments, complementary and alternative therapies, and CBT. Interestingly, the NHS website offers links to other organisations offering information and support. These organisations vary in style, content, and audience, so Women's Health Concern https://www.womens-health-concern.org/, as the patient-focused arm of the British Menopause Society, contains evidence-based factsheets on a range of topics. Menopause Matters https://www.menopausematters.co.uk/index.php also provides up-to-date and accurate information combined with a discussion forum where people can read and share questions, advice, and information amongst peers (see Chapter 6). The Daisy Network is aimed at women who have experienced premature menopause https://www.daisynetwork.org/ whilst Queermenopause https://www.queermenopause.com/resources contains resources for people going through the menopause who identify as LGBTQ+. Finally, there is a link to Menopause Café https://www.menopausecafe.net/ which provides information on place-based meet-ups for women seeking information and support.

All of the websites linked from the NHS website are UK oriented and focus on evidence-based or peer-reviewed research and information. However, Table 2.1 shows that sponsored information on Google can take people to pay for clinics or to information that may not be relevant to UK searchers. Whilst there has been a recent push to ensure that women are provided with correct and trusted information (Briggs et al., 2023), women use a wide range of other websites, online articles, and blogs as well as social media (see Chapter 5). How do we know what people are searching for in terms of online health about menopause, which resources do they select and engage with, and how do they make decisions about whether to trust it?

2.2 Trusting Online Information and Advice

Over the last 20 years, we have increased our understanding of how individuals search for, select, and evaluate online health advice and information. We also have a clearer idea of what factors are important in helping people decide whether to trust the information online. Our work on trust in online health information (Sillence et al., 2007a; Sillence & Briggs, 2015) provides support for a three-stage model of trust. First, individuals engage in rapid heuristic processing of information, efficiently sifting and rejecting sites they do not trust primarily on the basis of design features affecting the look and feel of the site. Participants then select sites for systematic evaluation, and here the credibility of the information is considered in terms of perceived expertise and absence of bias. Finally, some participants engage in a longer-term trusting relationship with the website, disclosing personal information. Overall, we see the importance of visual design clues to the appropriateness and ultimately the credibility of websites, followed by an in-depth evaluation of their content, noting the expertise, the currency, and the completeness of the information. A systematic review published in 2017 (Sbaffi & Rowley, 2017) noted that website design, clear layout, and interactive features have a positive effect on trust or credibility, whereas advertising has a negative effect. With regard to content features, authority of the author, ease of use, and currency have a positive effect on trust or credibility formation. A series of large-scale studies conducted over the last 20 years have charted the important factors predicting trust in online health information and advice (Harris et al., 2011; Sillence et al., 2019; Sillence, Branley-Bell, et al., 2025). These studies have shown a set of consistent findings around the importance of perceived impartiality, credible design, and quality information. A key feature of health websites that has changed over that period has been the inclusion of patient or personal experiences (PEx). The presence of PeX has steadily increased over the years, taking different forms (see Chapter 6) from forum posts, blogs and vlogs, and curated stories. Whilst PEx are liked they are not always trusted and in part that may come down to funding models (Sillence et al., 2013). Websites containing personal experiences can often feature advertising or sponsorship which many UK participants, at least, feel is incongruent with health information and advice.

2.3 A Closer Look at Menopause-Related Websites

In 2003, we asked 15 peri or post-menopausal women to search for and evaluate menopause information online (see Sillence et al., 2004; Sillence et al., 2007a for further details). They spent 30 minutes searching freely and then took part in a focus group to discuss the sites they had found and their thoughts on what makes a trustworthy resource. We found that women described the reasons for their quick rejection of sites in terms of poor design or an inappropriate look and feel to the sites. Pop-up adverts, non-intuitive names, and American spellings were all off-putting and caused participants to navigate away. Sites were chosen because of their unbiased content, their depth and breadth of information, and relevance for women like themselves (Sillence et al., 2004).

Since 2003, the landscape of online information has changed dramatically in terms of information providers, the technology, and the features of the sites (Sillence et al., 2007b). The context around menopause and menopause information has also changed. In 2003, the halting of the Women's Health Initiative (WHI) trial the previous year was still fresh in many women's minds. The discontinuation of the trial saw a concomitant decline in women starting and continuing their HRT. There followed a period of stabilisation and an increase in the number of women taking HRT from 2017 onwards (Sundell et al., 2023). In the UK, HRT prescriptions have risen 29% between 2022 and 2023 (NHS Business Services Authority, 2023) underpinned by national guidance, celebrity support, and the introduction of the HRT prepayment certificate that reduces the cost of HRT (British Menopause Society XE, 2021; NHS Business Services Authority, 2023; NICE, 2024).

More than twenty years after our 2003 study, we decided to look again at how peri and post-menopausal women search for and evaluate online menopause information and advice and how they decide which resources to trust and act upon. We asked 16 women to search online for 30 minutes for information and advice about menopause, and the websites they visited were automatically logged. We then carried out a semi-structured interview with all the women to ask them about the process of searching for menopause information and how they evaluated the information and the resources they encountered. We played back the screen recording so they could think aloud as they reviewed the sites they had visited, and we asked them to reflect upon their search strategies and what they wanted to get out of the information-seeking session. Finally, all the women took part in a focus group to share their thoughts and experiences of online menopause resources (see Sillence Osborne et al., 2026 for more details). Below we present two examples of participants' search strategies, an overview of the trust evaluations discussed by the participants during the focus groups, and finally an analysis of the sites visited.

2.3.1 Searching for Menopause Information Online

Women were asked to discuss their approach to searching for menopause information online. In the first example, 'Maria' talks about how she started her search in very general terms, and then clicked on different webpages of interest throughout her search. She did not have a specific question in mind.

> *I started with 'menopause' I think that's what I did. So I was looking up menopause in general you know general things about menopause, and it was the NHS website I looked at first. Then the recommended treatment was hormone replacement therapy so then I looked into that. Then, yeah, I found other articles about the disadvantages of that treatment. Then I looked up general things about menopause, for example, about age and different variables of why some women have it earlier than others but there is no consensus about that. Then I looked into how menopause affects mental health. That's where I was, I think. I look at the title first and then the little bit of content. Then I look to see if it's something that interests me. Some of them were very similar to what I have read before so I didn't click on it because I thought, "Well it's similar to what I read before." In terms of the HRT they say "Yes, talk to your doctor to see whether it's suitable for you." but it's [just very general]. It's actually suitable for most people and the advantages are better than the disadvantages. I thought, "Oh, there are disadvantages." Then you look into the other reporting, actually there are health consequences. According to that study, there were more disadvantages than advantages, apparent advantages. The only thing is that the possibility of bone fracture is less if you take hormone replacement therapy but you have more chance of getting cancer, heart disease, and some other stuff I don't remember. So, obviously, it's not as good as it seems so, yeah, it's interesting.*

In the second example, 'Alice' had a more specific question relating to ongoing symptoms.

> *So, I started with the question about whether you are perimenopausal, menopausal or post-menopausal trying to get an answer really, I still don't think I have an answer. If I am still getting symptoms in my 60 s what does that mean? So I started my search with that really. I just Googled and then started to go through those sites and there were so many other questions*

that people have asked, and they all pop up as well. I am not saying it's the best way but it's what I've always done. Anyway. So just playing around and stuff and... You know. I watched a video about- Well, she's a woman now, but she went through menopause when she was 10, and I didn't even know that was possible. So it was quite fascinating listening to what she said and I did quite a bit of it was actually quite productive, especially with regards to bio-identical HRT. I discovered some things to do with that as well.

2.3.2 Deciding whether or Not to Trust Menopause Information and Advice

The focus groups showed that women pick up on the design features of menopause websites and use this information to judge their tone and relevance. Participants thought that colour, for example, can convey either a medical or a more holistic approach to menopause. Familiar names and websites were important to women, with the NHS often being the first website visited. Websites that were linked from the NHS website were automatically trusted and seen as credible.

If it is linked to the NHS website, you think, 'oh, well, that must be a good resource to go to if they're...' It's almost like a recommendation isn't it, that it's there.

In line with this, there was a dislike of commercialisation on websites. Advertisements, particularly linked to pharmaceutical companies or any profit-based organisation, led to distrust of the information available on the website.

The top five or six [results] were ads for specific medications....so I avoided those kinds of things.

The relevance of the menopause information to each participant was essential, and overall, women discussed a specific lack of trust in sources that were not UK-based. Websites that referenced local offline groups or information were also welcomed, although sometimes difficult to find.

I was disappointed to see there was only one Menopause Café in the whole of North Manchester. So, oh, there might be one at [local place name] and then there was one in [local place name], but yeah so that made me think, "Oh well, it's not something that has really taken off," so I probably wouldn't go to the one in [local place name].

2.3.3 Menopause Websites

Our participants looked at between 5 and 17 sites (not counting search engines), and the mean number of sites was 9.875. One hundred and fifty two sites were logged (excluding search engines) and of those there were 84 unique sites. Nineteen of these sites were viewed by more than one participant. The NHS or NHS Inform (NHS in Scotland) website was viewed by all but two participants, Menopause Matters was viewed by 10 out of 16 participants, Balance by 7 of the participants, and the British Menopause Society by 6 participants. The sites viewed included academic journals, professional organisations, charities, private healthcare providers, retailers, and media outlets. A breakdown of the website types is shown in Table 2.2, and a more detailed description of the three top sites is shown in Table 2.3.

Our participants found menopause information on charity sites, professional body sites, in the media, and on private UK healthcare sites. These sites accounted for 36 out of 84 individual menopause sites visited. The range of websites from retail sites to the NHS to menopause advocacy groups and academic journals demonstrates the breadth of resources available, although the type of content and the depth of the information vary widely.

The top three sites visited by participants varied in terms of the type of website and the breadth and depth of content provided. All three sites covered the basics of menopause and described different symptoms. The breadth and depth of content on Menopause Matters and Balance were greater than on the NHS site, although the NHS site contained links to other websites for further information and support. Menopause Matters appears to be the most interactive resource with a peer support forum where people can exchange support and information, although

Table 2.2 Website types and examples

Website type	% of sites (N)	Example(s)
Charity	10.71 (9)	The menopause charity, Healthtalk
Professional bodies	10.71 (9)	Royal College of Obstetricians & Gynaecologists
Private UK healthcare	10.71 (9)	BUPA
Media	10.71 (9)	The telegraph
Web provider—Online health information	8.33 (7)	WebMD
Non-UK healthcare provider	7.14 (6)	HCA healthcare
Retail	5.95 (5)	Holland & Barrett
UK healthcare provider	4.76 (4)	NHS
Workplace support	4.76 (4)	NHS employers
Academic publications	4.76 (4)	Menopause journal
Menopause advocacy groups	3.57 (3)	Menopause support
Health and lifestyle apps	3.57 (3)	Clue
International organisation	2.38 (2)	WHO
Social networking sites	2.38 (2)	Mumsnet
Menopause coach/consultants	2.38 (2)	Menopause exchange
Blogs/individual run websites	2.38 (2)	Feisty menopause
Other	4.76 (4)	Tai chi

Balance contains personal stories from a diverse range of people. Balance has a comprehensive section on HRT, whilst the NHS and Menopause Matters contain more information on alternatives to HRT, including CBT, herbal remedies, and alternative therapies. Balance has a focus on inclusive menopause, highlighting the uniqueness of menopause with consideration for those experiencing early menopause, people with other health conditions, and vulnerable groups, and includes a consideration of age, gender, sexual identity, and ethnic background.

Table 2.3 Top three sites: NHS, Menopause Matters, Balance

		NHS	Menopause Matters	Balance
Website type		UK healthcare provider	Web provider	Private UK healthcare
Authorship		Unspecified	Named authors (HCPs)	HCPs
Menopause-related information	*Basic* (e.g. *what is menopause?)*	Definition, overview of symptoms, natural or surgical menopause	Definition and overview Information on diagnosis, premature menopause	Definition, extensive list of symptoms. Perimenopause covered
	Symptoms	Physical and mental health symptoms, changing periods	Early and late menopause symptoms and symptom questionnaire to complete and share with HCP	Extensive list of symptoms. Factsheets, podcasts, and videos relating to symptoms
	HRT	HRT explained Oestrogen Testosterone	HRT explained, risks and benefits, review process Decision tree	Comprehensive section on HRT
	Alternative treatments	CBT Non-hormonal medicines Complimentary treatments	CBT Aromatherapy acupuncture, yoga Phytoestrogens Herbal remedies	Anti-depressants CBT

(continued)

Table 2.3 (continued)

		NHS	Menopause Matters	Balance
	Lifestyle changes	Exercise Clothing Diet Relaxation	Exercise Diet Relaxation	Exercise Diet Relaxation and mindfulness
	Sex and relationships	Brief mention in relation to symptoms—Reduced sex drive, pain during sex	Mentioned in relation to vaginal problems and painful sex	Resources in the form of articles and links to balance podcasts
	Workplace	Brief mention of the potential impact in the overview section	Dedicated page with links to other articles and downloadable resources	Main tab on homepage—Large section of resources devoted to workplace
Community features	*Peer support forum* *Personal stories*	None	Peer support forum	Personal stories of menopause
Contact information	*Email*	None	Email addresses provided	Email addresses provided
Links to further information/access to references/ further information sources		Links to NHS and private specialists List of charities offering information and support	Links to BMS menopause specialist Links to magazine articles	Links to other resources including the balance app, podcasts, and related sites
Commercial features related to menopause (adverts or links to menopause-related products and services)	*Shop/products available to purchase* *Book a consultation or course*	None	Adverts supplied by Google not endorsed by MM	None Book a consultation

2.4 Discussion

Websites continue to be an important source of information and advice about menopause for women. Women have multiple sources of information online available to them, but seek familiar, trusted sites such as the NHS, at least as a starting point for their online information. Searching for information can be difficult, especially without a specific question in mind. Information can feel contradictory at times and often overwhelming. As in 2003, participants in our recent study were trying to find information that was relevant to them. The style and the tone of the information were important alongside the framing of menopause and the source of the information. Websites in 2024 are more interconnected than twenty years ago. Some websites allow women to book menopause consultations or promote sister apps or podcasts.

The range of organisations and individuals providing information and support on menopause is vast and diverse. This is not simply an online landscape dominated by healthcare organisations and providers. Retail, media, coaches, and consultants, as well as charities and professional bodies, provide a potentially overwhelming mix of content for women (Sillence, Osborne, et al., 2026). Popular websites appear to provide at least the basic information on menopause symptoms and treatments, with some detailing some of the less well-covered topics such as menopause and the workplace and sex, relationships, and menopause.

All our participants relied upon the Google search facility to find the websites. This study was carried before the Artificial Intelligence (AI) overview for Google become widely available. Given how many women started with the first few hits, it would be interesting to explore the role of AI in signalling trustworthy and credible information to women, and whilst this will be explored further in Chapter 7, it is useful to briefly touch upon this topic here. Early reviews of online health information focused on the quality and readability of the information being served up to individuals (Eysenbach et al., 2002). With the advent of consumer accessible AI, the question of quality in terms of accuracy and readability is heavily foregrounded in research once again. Studies assessing the quality of information and appropriateness of ChatGPT responses for patients show variation in terms of reading levels and accuracy (Cocci et al., 2024). For sensitive health topics, a conversational agent may be a useful way of accessing relevant health information, although they may produce more complex and less accessible answers to health-related enquiries than Google searches (Burns et al., 2024), and they vary considerably between AI chatbots (Mondal et al., 2025). Accessibility and quality are important factors for women when accessing any kind of menopause resource (Emter & Chavula, 2025), and this is likely to remain the case when using AI to seek menopause information.

References

Briggs, P., Hamoda, H., Rymer, J., Morris, E., & Moger, S. (2023). Menopause care for women: Supporting the NHS to support women. *Post Reproductive Health, 29*(1), 4–5.

British Menopause Society (2021). BMS & WHC's 2020 recommendations on hormone replacement therapy in menopausal women March 2021 https://thebms.org.uk/publications/consensus-statements/bms-whcs-2020-recommendations-on-hormone-replacement-therapy-in-menopausal-women/

Burns, C., Bakaj, A., Berishaj, A., Hristidis, V., Deak, P., & Equils, O. (2024). Use of generative AI for improving health literacy in reproductive health: Case study. *JMIR Formative Research, 8, Article e59434*.

Cocci, A., Pezzoli, M., Lo Re, M., Russo, G. I., Asmundo, M. G., Fode, M., et al. (2024). Quality of information and appropriateness of ChatGPT outputs for urology patients. *Prostate Cancer and Prostatic Diseases, 27*(1), 103–108.

Davies, E., & Halliday, V. (2025). Nutrition information and the menopause: An online survey of perimenopausal and menopausal women. *Post Reproductive Health, 31*(2), 65–72.

Emter, F., & Chavula, C. (2025, March). Seeking control: How women evaluate and use menopause related information. *Proceedings of the 2025 ACM SIGIR Conference on Human Information Interaction and Retrieval* (pp. 179–194).

Eysenbach, G., Powell, J., Kuss, O., & Sa, E. R. (2002). Empirical studies assessing the quality of health information for consumers on the world wide web. *JAMA 287*(20), 2691. https://doi.org/10.1001/jama.287.20.2691

Harper, J. C., Phillips, S., Biswakarma, R., Yasmin, E., Saridogan, E., Radhakrishnan, S., & Talaulikar, V. (2022). An online survey of perimenopausal women to determine their attitudes and knowledge of the menopause. Women's Health, 18, Article 17455057221106890.

Harris, P. R., Sillence, E., & Briggs, P. (2011). Perceived threat and corroboration: Key factors that improve a predictive model of trust in internet-based health information and advice. Journal of Medical Internet Research, 13(3), Article e51.

Lupton, D., & Maslen, S. (2019). How women use digital technologies for health: Qualitative interview and focus group study. Journal of Medical Internet Research, 21(1), Article e11481.

Mondal, H., Tiu, D. N., Mondal, S., Dutta, R., Naskar, A., & Podder, I. (2025). Evaluating accuracy and readability of responses to midlife health questions: A comparative analysis of six large language model chatbots. *Journal of Mid-life Health, 16*(1), 45–50.

Munn, C., Vaughan, L., Talaulikar, V., Davies, M. C., & Harper, J. C. (2022). Menopause knowledge and education in women under 40: Results from an online survey. Women's Health, 18, Article 17455057221139660.

NHS Business Services Authority. (2023). Hormone replacement therapy: England April 2015 to June 2023. https://www.nhsbsa.nhs.uk/statistical-collections/hormone-replacement-therapy-england/hormone-replacement-therapy-england-april-2015-june-2023

NICE (2024). Menopause: diagnosis and management. NICE guideline [NG23] Published: 12 November 2015. Last updated: 07 November 2024. https://www.nice.org.uk/guidance/ng23

Sbaffi, L., & Rowley, J. (2017). Trust and credibility in web-based health information: A review and agenda for future research. Journal of Medical Internet Research, 19(6), Article e218.

Sillence, E., Blythe, J. M., Briggs, P., & Moss, M. (2019). A revised model of trust in internet-based health information and advice: Cross-sectional questionnaire study. *Journal of Medical Internet Research, 21*(11), e11125.

Sillence, E., Branley-Bell, D., Moss, M., & Briggs, P. (2025). A model of trust in online COVID-19 information and advice: Cross-sectional questionnaire study. JMIR Infodemiology, 5(1), Article e59317.

Sillence, E., & Briggs, P. (2015). Trust and engagement in online health: A timeline approach. In S. S. Sundar (Ed.), *The handbook of the psychology of communication technology* (pp. 469–487). Wiley Blackwell.

Sillence, E., Briggs, P., Fishwick, L., & Harris, P. (2004, April). Trust and mistrust of online health sites. *Proceedings of the SIGCHI Conference on Human Factors in Computing Systems*, 663–670.

Sillence, E., Briggs, P., Harris, P., & Fishwick, L. (2007b). Health websites that people can trust—The case of hypertension. *Interacting with Computers, 19*(1), 32–42.

Sillence, E., Briggs, P., Harris, P. R., & Fishwick, L. (2007a). How do patients evaluate and make use of online health information? *Social Science & Medicine, 64*(9), 1853–1862.

Sillence, E., Hardy, C., & Briggs, P. (2013, May). Why don't we trust health websites that help us help each other? An analysis of online peer-to-peer healthcare. *Proceedings of the 5th Annual ACM Web Science Conference*, 396–404.

Sillence, E., Osborne, A. K., Claisse, C., & Durrant, A. C. (2026). Understanding the challenges of using digital health technologies for menopause information. Patient Education and Counseling, Article 109375.

Sundell, M., Brynhildsen, J., Holm, A. C. S., Fredrikson, M., & Hoffmann, M. (2023). Trends in the incidence, prevalence and sales volume of menopausal hormone therapy in Sweden from 2000 to 2021. Maturitas, 175, Article 107787.

Tariq, B., Phillips, S., Biswakarma, R., Talaulikar, V., & Harper, J. C. (2023). Women's knowledge and attitudes to the menopause: A comparison of women over 40 who were in the perimenopause, post menopause and those not in the peri or post menopause. BMC Women's Health, 23(1), Article 460.

3

Menopause Apps

Abstract Mobile health applications (mHealth) are increasingly popular and provide information and interactive features to support people with their health and wellbeing. Women's health is a growing market with apps for menstrual health, fertility and pregnancy, and more recently menopause. This chapter explores the role of smartphone apps in menopause support and is organised as follows: We (1) introduce the rise of mHealth in women's health and menopause specifically and provide an overview of menopause apps and their features. We then (2) highlight some of the current discussion points around the promotion and use of mHealth in women's health. The next section (3) details findings from a series of studies looking at menopause apps, drawing examples from our own research looking at women's experiences of using menopause apps. These studies show how women are using the different features of the apps to support their menopause journeys and highlight the role of HCP integration. The final section (4) draws together the literature and presents conclusions and considerations for future research.

Keywords mHealth apps · Symptom tracking · Women's health · Healthcare professional communication · Patient empowerment

E. Sillence and A. Osborne, *Digital Health Technologies and the Menopause*, Palgrave Studies in Cyberpsychology, https://doi.org/10.1007/978-3-032-25909-7_3

3.1 Mhealth, Women's Health, and Menopause

Mobile health applications (mHealth apps) provide a resource across a range of women's health issues, including pregnancy and parenting (Brown et al., 2019; Lupton & Pedersen, 2016), menstrual tracking and menstrual pain (Levy & Romo-Avilés, 2019; Trépanier et al., 2023), and fertility (Ali et al., 2021; Miner et al., 2022). Whilst researchers have noted the variability in the quality of the apps and the information provided (Brown et al., 2019), user studies have highlighted benefits including increased knowledge and reassurance (Lupton & Pedersen, 2016). Using mHealth apps also brings challenges. Checking the validity of app-based information is effortful, as is the process of tracking personal health data, and, in some cases, it can prove distressing (Levy & Romo-Avilés, 2019).

Menopause apps vary considerably in their functionality and features. They may differ in their overall purpose, for example, to act as a diary or self-assessment guide or an informational resource (Gkrozou et al., 2019). Basic apps may contain information and/or a period tracking function, whereas more advanced menopause apps often contain multiple tracking features including menstrual cycle, menopause symptoms, and symptom triggers. These apps may allow users to visualise their data and print off reports for HCPs and have community or peer chat features (Sillence et al., 2023).

There are a relatively small number of reviews of menopause apps focusing predominantly on the features, quality, and authorship of the apps. Gkrozou et al. (2019), for example, noted that few apps had HCP input into their content, and many apps receive mixed ratings and recommendations from experts as well as women and users themselves (Greffin et al., 2025). Paripoorani et al. (2023) carried out a review of menopause apps with an emphasis on osteoporosis. Using validated measures, they noted that the average quality score of the reviewed apps was 3.1 out of 5 and the mean functionality score was 4.57 out of 11. The authors suggested that more expert input was desirable to improve menopause apps.

3.1.1 Menopause Apps and their Features

In our review of menopause apps (see Sillence et al., 2023), we wanted to get a better understanding of the variability of the apps available and focused on the overall quality of the apps alongside their features. We also noted that many of the apps reviewed in Gkrozou et al. (2019) no longer existed, indicating the transience of the app market. Table 3.1 shows an overview of the different features we noted in our review. A small number of the apps reviewed only contained basic menopause information—these apps were not interactive and did not contain any tracking features. Most apps contained more features whilst a small group of apps contained a wide range of features, including tracking, data visualisations, and tailored content. A number of apps contained community features such as curated stories or access to peer support forums for exchanging information and advice.

The most popular apps, in terms of number of downloads, contained a wider range of features, whilst less popular apps contained relatively few features. More popular apps had higher mean quality scores as measured by the well-used Mobile App Rating Scale (MARS Stoyanov et al., 2015). Those apps that explicitly stated they had HCP input and support also had a MARS mean quality score of above 4, indicating good quality. Table 3.2 provides a descriptive account of a popular 'feature-rich' menopause app alongside a less popular 'information-only' app. Comparing these apps, it is clear that the popular app contains a range of engaging features alongside well-referenced, updated articles, whilst the less popular app contains basic menopause information that is commonly found within other apps and on other websites. The apps compared in Table 3.2 were reviewed as part of Sillence et al. (2023), although when we updated the information for this chapter, we noted that some apps no longer existed (Menopausal)—once again highlighting the volatility of the mobile health app environment (Larsen et al., 2016).

Whilst reviews of apps have highlighted issues with quality and limited HCP involvement, there is limited research focusing on menopause app users themselves. An exception is Andrews et al. (2023), who demonstrated that using menopause apps can be effective in reducing menopausal symptoms but less is known about how women come to use

Table 3.1 Features of menopause apps

Overall feature	Description of feature	Details and examples
Tailored set-up	Users can personalise their interaction with app	Input personal details to complete personalised set-up
Information	Menopause-related information	Basics (e.g. what is menopause?) Symptoms Overview of treatments including sections on hormone replacement Therapy (HRT) and alternative treatments Diet and exercise Sex and relationships Workplace
Tracking	Users can track their personal health and lifestyle data	Symptoms of menopause, e.g. and symptom triggers Menstrual cycle tracking Medication
Review and report	Users can visualise their tracked data and create reports	Visualise symptoms, symptom triggers, or menstrual cycle over time in chart format Generate a summary report to keep or share with a healthcare professional
Community	Users can read and share peer-generated content	Forum that allows users to read and post messages Curated stories for users to read and option to submit experiences of menopause
Interactive elements	Interactive polls, experiments with feedback	Audio guides and self-help Exercise challenges Experiments Polls Calculators, e.g. BMI, calories

(continued)

Table 3.1 (continued)

Overall feature	Description of feature	Details and examples
Links to further information	Access to references/ further information sources	References provided for information, including links to academic articles Links to YouTube videos
Contact information	Contact details for app developers	Email address for contacting developers Encouragement to contact or feedback to developers Links to social media presence
Commercial features related to menopause	Adverts or links to menopause-related products and services	Link to purchase menopause-related products Link to book a consultation with a menopause specialist or coach or register for a menopause-related course

Table 3.2 Description of a popular and a less popular menopause app

Balance
Description: Balance is a popular menopause app with over one million downloads and a review star rating of 4.7 (Play Store September 2025).
Number of reviews: (android) 45 K reviews
Created by: Dr. Louise Newson
Features: Bespoke articles with references, tracking and data visualisations, community features, polls and interactive content.
Pricing: Free to download, premium paid for content.
Menopausal
Description: A very basic app providing basic information on menopause. Very few downloads (10) and no user reviews (September 2021). Content is replicated on other menopause apps.
Created by: Unknown
Features: Basic information on menopause only.

menopause apps in the first place, the way they engage with the functionality and the wider impact, if any, the apps have on their menopause journey.

In the absence of user studies, critiques of the narratives surrounding women's health apps provide an interesting starting point. Critics have argued that menopause apps and other FemTech technologies such as period and fertility trackers purport to offer women a range of empowering features whilst actually reinforcing sexist stereotypes and diminishing women's credibility as people who can 'trust their own experiences and gather reliable knowledge about their own bodies' (Hendl & Jansky, 2022). We note the researchers call for further research into users' actual experiences of 'empowerment' (Hendl & Jansky, 2022) and epistemic injustice and their experiences of using FemTech.

3.1.2 Women's Experiences of Smartphone Apps for Menopause

To better understand women's experiences of using menopause apps, we report data from two of our studies focusing on recent or current app users.

In the first (Sillence et al., 2023), we examined the features of 18 menopause apps, rated the apps using the MARS (Stoyanov et al., 2015) and undertook a thematic analysis of 551 written reviews. Reviews that referenced the functionality of the app or included details about how the app affected menopause experiences were analysed using an inductive reflexive thematic analysis approach (Braun & Clarke, 2021). Reviews of apps were positive in nature and led to the development of four themes: 'empowering functions', 'I'm not alone', 'function wish list', and 'usability and privacy'.

The theme *'empowering functions'* showed how the users felt empowered by using the features of the smartphone apps. Empowerment corresponded with increased understanding of menopause and an increased sense of legitimacy. Empowerment was also related to increased confidence in interactions with healthcare professionals. User reviews documented the importance of being able to share reports with HCPs, but also the role of apps in allowing users to read more widely on menopause to consolidate knowledge and to enhance sense-making.

The theme *'I'm not alone'* is related to the sense of support and connection users felt with the wider community. Users felt a sense of being close to others going through 'similar experiences' but also recognised the wider community around menopause, for example, healthcare professionals and app developers, especially when those developers were women. Users commented on the sense of connection with peers through community features on apps and valued reading other people's experiences and asking their own questions.

The theme *'function wish list'* captured users' desire to increase the personalisation of the app to meet their individual menopause needs. Users wanted more options for capturing their symptoms and symptom triggers and greater control over how and when they recorded information. They expressed a desire to work with developers by providing feedback to improve apps.

The theme *'usability and privacy'* highlighted concerns over the collection and sharing of personal data. Participants were not always happy to set up accounts, especially when it was not clear as to why this was necessary or how their data would be used or possibly shared. Users queried why certain pieces of personal data were being collected, for example, telephone numbers, and noted problems accessing privacy statements. Concerns around technical problems and glitches undermined faith in the app.

In our second study (Sillence Osborne Kemp & McKellar, 2025), we gathered qualitative data from women who were using or had used menopause apps in the past to explore some of the themes emerging from the reviews.

We collected qualitative responses from 29 women to a series of online open-ended questions about their experiences of using menopause apps. Ten of these women also took part in a follow-up interview where we explored their experiences in more detail. We asked women about their motivations for using the app, what they thought of the experience of interacting with the app, how their app use had varied, and how they thought the app had impacted their menopause experience, if at all.

We found that most women had come to the app through a personal recommendation from a friend or colleague or because they had heard the app mentioned on another platform, e.g. on Instagram or in the mainstream media. Overall, most people thought that apps were easy to use and particularly valued the tracking and community elements and less so the information. Menopause information was often sought via websites (Chapter 2), and women often used multiple digital resources to support their menopause journey.

Here we summarise the ways in which women described how menopause apps supported their menopause experiences. Menopause apps positively support menopause experiences in two main ways: By facilitating a better, more holistic understanding of menopause as it affects the individual and by underpinning better communication with healthcare professionals around menopause.

Better Understanding of Menopause; Feeling Normal and Not Alone

Women used apps to gain a comprehensive picture of their unique menopause experience. This involved finding out about symptoms linked to menopause and then relating their experiences to 'normal' issues supported by the sense that they were 'not alone'.

For many women, using the apps to track symptoms was the first time they realised that some of the symptoms they were experiencing were menopause related rather than standalone.

> *And what I found what I found really surprising with it was so many of the things I was experiencing were on this list that and it was like, whoa, I didn't know that was to do with my menopause. I didn't know it.*

Realising that certain symptoms were part of their menopause experience helped women normalise their experiences. The apps helped provide reassurance that symptoms were explainable and that other women were experiencing similar issues.

> *It makes me realise that it is "normal" the symptoms I'm experiencing.*

Using the apps prompted some women to seek coping strategies and think about treatment options. Some of the women talked about finding perspective in relation to menopause and taking control of their lives and the more subtle role that apps could play in that process.

> *[I was looking] for a better understanding of not what was happening, but why it's happening and I found once I understand why I'm good with that, I think OK, this is happening because of this and that's fine.*

Recording and Tracking to Present Evidence and Have Better Conversations with HCPs

Apps played a role for some women in pushing back against the difficulties they reported in accessing the information and support they sought regarding menopause and access to HRT. Apps helped women feel better able to have meaningful discussions with HCPs.

Some women reported protracted difficulties with their HCPs. Women were looking for advice and support, but often found it difficult to get the recognition they needed in the first place.

> *I know GPs are busy, but they don't seem to like to listen, I told them I know my own body. I was trying to prove to them that I was going through the menopause cause they didn't seem to believe me.*

Women explained how using the app had proved important in terms of providing 'proof' about their menopause symptoms, their severity, and duration. Women described taking the app to show the HCP the data visualisations of the tracked symptoms or menstrual cycle, and that this was part of the empowering function of apps. Through the app, women felt they were in a much better place to tell their story and to present a clear and concise account of their menopause experience to others.

> *I do think they help women advocate for themselves by learning and understanding what's going on with their bodies in order to feel confident and empowered to speak to health professionals, employers and peers.*

The Potential Downsides of Using Menopause Apps

Across our two studies, the benefits of using menopause apps were overwhelming; however, some women did highlight the potential challenges in using menopause apps as well.

Some users in the reviews pointed to limitations in the way the apps allowed them to enter their data. Users wanted to be able to customise the types of data they could collect and the ways in which they could capture it. Other reviewers had concerns about the privacy and security of the data and questioned why apps needed to collect the data they did.

> *I will be deleting this because it appears you are required to create an account to use this. I want it only for my personal tracking, I don't want to share any information with anyone.*

These usability and privacy concerns were less prevalent in our second study, although app users did think it was important to know the 'person behind the app' or preferred to have had the app recommended to them. Most of our app users thought they would not have entered any personal details into the app if they had not known who was behind the app. The fact that the Balance app was 'owned' by Dr. Louise Newson and that she was an HCP, cross-referenced by other menopause celebrities and was familiar to them from her TV appearances, helped in terms of the app's credibility.

Some women found the information on the apps quite minimal in relation to web-based resources or to non-digital sources such as menopause books, and many women indicated that once they started HRT, they no longer used the app.

3.1.3 Discussion

Overall, menopause apps are viewed positively, providing access to information, peer support, and perhaps most usefully to tracking and monitoring features. It is these features which set apps apart from other digital technologies for menopause and these features that women typically evoke when explaining how important the app has been in terms of empowerment. In our studies, we saw women describe the empowering function of apps to better understand their menopause and to facilitate better conversations about menopause with their HCPs. That digital technologies are empowering for women is not a given within the literature and requires further scrutiny (see Chapter 7). Suffice to say women's own experiences suggested that apps had played some positive role in relation to their menopause journey.

We still know very little about how healthcare professionals feel about menopause apps and their patients using these apps and sharing their data visualisations. In one of our studies, a participant told us that her doctor had advised her to download and use an app to track her symptoms. It transpired that the doctor was using the app herself. Aside from this example, we know that HCPs are wary of patients using their own devices for tracking health data. User error and device reliability are potential barriers to acceptance, along with the additional pressures on consultation times (Tomasella & Morgan, 2021; West et al., 2016). Engaging with tracking data can place a burden on HCPs, but raising awareness about women's use of menopause apps and having those conversations early could provide an opportunity to signpost to more accurate, usable, and reliable apps.

Tracking and recording personal health data on apps and other devices is not without its downsides. Studies have shown the burden on patients through poorly designed apps that impede use, privacy, and security concerns and difficulties over how to interpret data (Peng et al., 2016; Schroeder et al., 2018). App abandonment is commonplace (de Boer et al., 2023; Larsen et al., 2016), and there can be considerable overlap between apps so that women already tracking their menstrual cycles on a fitness app may not want the additional burden of having to track cycles on a menopause app. Again, conversations with HCPs about how tracking might fit with existing health practices would be beneficial here.

For many people, apps may be more convenient, but the process of journaling and tracking is not confined to the digital realm. Claisse et al. (2022) found that paper diaries held value for people practising self-care and raised the concern that translating the diaries into a digital format might detract from the 'therapeutic-ness' of the diary. Brown et al. (2022) also captured participants' non-digital practices for recording personal health data. The authors noted highly personal forms of recording and reflecting changes in, for example, mood, including drawing shapes and doodles, and these were not always designed to be shared with others.

Our studies have indicated that many people were focused on exploring and getting access to HRT when using the apps. For many, their app use ended once they had started their treatment. Whilst this could be a limitation of the recruitment approach in our studies, it would be interesting to see how people respond to the development of apps that foreground other forms of treatment and self-care. Currently, some popular apps have a strong focus on HRT, and there is space within app development for more holistic approaches to menopause advice and support.

Finally, menopause app use is still in its infancy. The landscape of menopause apps means that comparing across time points is difficult. Apps change, develop, stop working, or cease to exist. The nature of the app market means that many apps come and go, and it is difficult to compare apps over time or to witness the evolution of the resource. The funding model also poses challenges for women who find that more useful or extensive content is behind a subscription paywall. Understanding how women use menopause apps over time and their changing experiences in relation to the resource is an important line of research. Access to many more personalised features is often limited by cost, and understanding how these features could prove useful in supporting menopause experiences has not yet been explored.

References

Ali, R., Gürtin, Z. B., & Harper, J. C. (2021). Do fertility tracking applications offer women useful information about their fertile window? *Reproductive Biomedicine Online, 42*(1), 273–281.

Andrews, R., Lancastle, D., Bache, K., & Lacey, A. S. (2023). Does health and her app use improve menopausal symptoms? A longitudinal cohort study. *BMJ Open, 13*(12), Article e077185.

Braun, V., & Clarke, V. (2021). *Thematic analysis: A practical guide* (1st ed.), Sage Publications.

Brown, H. M., Bucher, T., Collins, C. E., Rollo, M. E., McCaffrey, T. A., & Sze, K. (2019). A review of pregnancy iPhone apps assessing their quality, inclusion of behaviour change techniques, and nutrition information. *Maternal and Child Nutrition, 15*(3), Article e12768.

Brown, R., Sillence, E., Coventry, L., & Bell, S. (2022). Understanding the attitudes and experiences of people living with potentially stigmatised long-term health conditions with respect to collecting and sharing health and lifestyle data. *DIGITAL HEALTH, 8*, 1–16.

Claisse, C., Kasadha, B., Stumpf, S., & Durrant, A. C. (2022, April). Investigating daily practices of self-care to inform the design of supportive health technologies for living and ageing well with HIV. *Proceedings of the 2022 CHI Conference on Human Factors in Computing Systems* (pp. 1–19).

de Boer, M., Hendriks, M., Krahmer, E., & Moors, A. (2023). *Un-tracking menopause: How not using self-tracking technologies mediates women's self-experiences in menopause* (p. 13634593231204171). Health.

Gkrozou, F., Tsonis, O., Godden, M., Siafaka, V., & Paschopoulos, M. (2019). Mobile health (mHealth) apps focused on menopause: Are they any good? *Post Reproductive Health, 25*(4), 191–198.

Greffin, K., Muehlmann, M., Pauleikhoff, A., Stelling, B., Muehlan, H., Stach, M., Heesen, C., & Tomczyk, S. (2025). *Embracing change: Navigating menopause with the help of mobile health apps in Germany* (p. 100320). Comprehensive Psychoneuroendocrinology.

Hendl, T., & Jansky, B. (2022). Tales of self-empowerment through digital health technologies: A closer look at 'Femtech'. *Review of Social Economy, 80*(1), 29–57.

Larsen, M. E., Nicholas, J., & Christensen, H. (2016). Quantifying app store dynamics: Longitudinal tracking of mental health apps. *JMIR mHealth and uHealth, 4*(3), Article e96.

Levy, J., & Romo-Avilés, N. (2019). "a good little tool to get to know yourself a bit better": A qualitative study on users' experiences of app-supported menstrual tracking in Europe. *BMC Public Health, 19*, 1–11.

Lupton, D., & Pedersen, S. (2016). An Australian survey of women's use of pregnancy and parenting apps. *Women and Birth, 29*(4), 368–375.

Miner, S. A., Gelgoot, E. N., Lahuec, A., Bui, J., Willis, A. R., & Chan, C. (2022). "who needs an app? Fertility patients' use of a novel mobile health app". *Digital Health, 8*.

Paripoorani, D., Gasteiger, N., Hawley-Hague, H., Scott, H., Booth, A., Godfrey, A., & Todd, C. (2023). A systematic review of menopause apps with an emphasis on osteoporosis. *BMC Women's Health, 23*(1), Article 518.

Peng, W., Kanthawala, S., Yuan, S., & Hussain, S. A. (2016). A qualitative study of user perceptions of mobile health apps. *BMC public health, 16*(1), article 1158.

Schroeder, J., Chung, C. F., Epstein, D. A., Karkar, R., Parsons, A., Murinova, N., Chung, J., & Munson, S. A. (2018, June). Examining self-tracking by people with migraine: Goals, needs, and opportunities in a chronic health condition. *Proceedings of the 2018 designing interactive systems conference* (pp. 135–148).

Sillence, E., Hardy, C., & Kemp, E. (2023). "this app just gets me": Assessing the quality, features and user reviews of menopause smartphone apps. *Journal of Consumer Health On The Internet, 27*(2), 156–172.

Sillence, E., Osborne, A. K., Kemp, E., & McKellar, K. (2025). Menopause apps: Personal health tracking, empowerment and epistemic injustice. *Digital Health, 11,* Article 20552076251330782.

Stoyanov, S. R., Hides, L., Kavanagh, D. J., Zelenko, O., Tjondronegoro, D., & Mani, M. (2015). Mobile app rating scale: A new tool for assessing the quality of health mobile apps. *JMIR mHealth and uHealth, 3,* (1), Article e3422.

Tomasella, F., & Morgan, H. M. (2021). "Sometimes I don't have a pulse… and I'm still alive!" interviews with healthcare professionals to explore their experiences of and views on population-based digital health technologies. *DIGITAL HEALTH, 7,* 20552076211018366.

Trépanier, L. C., Lamoureux, É., Bjornson, S. E., Mackie, C., Alberts, N. M., & Gagnon, M. M. (2023). Smartphone apps for menstrual pain and symptom management: A scoping review. *Internet Interventions, 31,* Article 100605.

West, P., Giordano, R., Van Kleek, M., & Shadbolt, N. (2016, May). The quantified patient in the doctor's office: Challenges & opportunities. In *Proceedings of the 2016 chi conference on human factors in computing systems* (pp. 3066-3078).

4

The Role of Podcasts in Menopause Communication

Abstract Podcasts are an increasingly popular platform allowing users to engage with information in a wider range of places, for example, in their homes, cars, or when out for a run. We know that podcasts can be an effective learning tool for healthcare trainees in women's health (Dmytryshyn & Selk, 2022), but less is known about their potential for supporting women going through menopause. The audio format of the platform offers an interesting opportunity to explore engagement with menopause information and other women's experiences. However, relatively little is known about the accessibility and engagement of this format, with the notable exception of Edwards et al. (2021) who found women engaged favourably with the podcast 'menopause unmuted'. In this chapter, we (1) Introduce podcasts and provide an overview of the menopause podcast landscape noting key podcast series and topics and (2) Present some findings from our recent work exploring women's preferences and experiences engaging with menopause information via podcasts focusing on how women find and select relevant podcasts, where and when they engage with format, and how they evaluate the information they encounter. We then reflect on the format itself and discuss how the distinct features of the resource may present specific opportunities to users.

E. Sillence and A. Osborne, *Digital Health Technologies and the Menopause*, Palgrave Studies in Cyberpsychology, https://doi.org/10.1007/978-3-032-25909-7_4

Keywords Podcasts · Audio health information · Narrative engagement · Accessibility · Menopause communication · Parasocial relationships

4.1 What Are Podcasts and How Do People Engage With Them?

Podcasts are one of the newer uses of internet technology to disseminate information (Robinson & Ritzko, 2009). They are digital audio recordings available online, often with the ability to download and listen offline. Like television shows, there are podcast episodes and series, and they offer a wide variety of content and programming, including news, information, interviews, and stories to select and listen to on demand (Tobin & Guadagno, 2022). Podcasts are highly accessible through several mainstream platforms such as Spotify, Apple Podcasts, Google Podcasts, and BBC Sounds. Recent years have seen a rise in the popularity of podcasts. From survey studies, we know that about 20% of participants surveyed reported having used a podcast (Harper et al., 2022), and over 20% of UK adults are now listening to at least one podcast a week, with 37% listening to health and wellbeing podcasts (Ofcom, 2024).

These episodic digital audio recordings have the "capacity to reach people in their homes, cars, and offices" (Harter, 2019, p. 126), ensuring information remains accessible and convenient. A significant feature of podcasts is the ability to listen whilst carrying out other activities. Perks et al. (2019), for example, found that people often perform mundane tasks whilst listening to podcasts, such as commuting or cleaning and other household activities. Podcasts are also often made for smaller audiences than traditional media (Verdusco, 2016) and can therefore be more detailed and specific in their topic areas. Research has indicated that podcasts can be used as a tool to communicate and promote health information, health-related behaviours, increase knowledge, and impact wellbeing (LaBrosse & Albrecht, 2013; Robins et al., 2024; Turner-McGrievy et al., 2013) across a range of topics including menopause

(Edwards et al., 2021). These may focus on medical education, nutrition, fitness, and peer support.

4.2 Podcasts for Health and Menopause Information

Increasingly, this audio format is being utilised for the purpose of educating on health topics (e.g. Elilnesan et al., 2025; Kelly et al., 2022; Militello et al., 2021). Podcasts have the potential to simplify complex health topics and provide multiple perspectives to ensure the relatability of the content to the listener. The accessibility and convenience of podcasts make them valuable tools for disseminating this health information (Robins et al., 2024). The audio nature of podcasts can provide an alternative way to digest health information, and a small body of research has found that general health information presented in this way can increase health knowledge (e.g. Krawczyk et al., 2012; Ross et al., 2010), more than written content (Armstrong et al., 2011). However, only a few papers have specifically considered this in relation to menopause (e.g. Edwards et al., 2021; Shaw et al., 2022). We know that podcasts can be an effective learning tool for healthcare trainees in women's health (Dmytryshyn & Selk, 2022), but less is known about their potential for supporting women going through menopause.

The content and availability of menopause-specific podcasts is vast and has continued to rise in recent years, with both podcast series dedicated to the topic as well as individual episodes from other lifestyle series. Hundreds, if not thousands, of podcasts are dedicated to menopause discussions across multiple platforms. The Dr. Louise Newson podcast, for example, has over 300 episodes (as of October 2025).

In our recent study, we asked 16 women to listen to menopause podcasts for a minimum of two hours over a two-week period (see Sillence et al., 2025). The aim was to explore how women engage with podcasts as a means of accessing digital menopause information and to understand their information needs. Participants were asked to record which podcast episodes they listened to; 74 podcast episodes were documented from 22 different podcast series. The top five podcast series listened to by participants were The Dr. Louise Newson Podcast, Thriving in Menopause, The Happy Menopause Podcast, Menopause Matters, and It Can't Just Be Me. Our participants reported listening to episodes on diverse topics, including brain fog and dementia, perimenopause anxiety, hypnotherapy, HRT, relationships, work and nutrition, and menopause and exercise. Within a podcast series, participants were able to engage with medical-based information, holistic, alternative solutions, sharing stories and self-help tips. Participants approached the task by searching for a podcast series and then looking through the episode titles to choose which one to listen to.

> *I listened to podcasts on Spotify. I initially did a search for menopause podcasts via the Spotify search function, and it gave numerous hits. I chose the first one on perimenopause anxiety based on my own feelings of anxiety which have only really happened since being perimenopausal*

Nearly all the participants were unfamiliar with using podcasts prior to the study, and those who were familiar were new to menopause-based podcasts. However, the experience of engaging with podcasts was extensively positive, with some participants being surprised about the podcasts and how informative they were:

> *I found the episodes I listened to very engaging. I have not really considered listening to podcasts on the topics previously and was positively surprised how informative the podcasts were*

4.3 Why Engage With Podcasts over Other Digital Health Technologies?

The main motivation for women engaging with any digital health technology for menopause information is to learn about the menopause experience (Osborne & Sillence, 2025), and this is also true for podcasts specifically (Edwards et al., 2021). Most of our participants enjoyed engaging with the podcasts despite many being unfamiliar with or even sceptical about the format prior to the study. So why might people choose to engage with podcasts over other digital health technologies?

Previous research has highlighted that individuals engage with and absorb health information to a greater extent when the communication strategy used is entertaining (Busselle & Bilandzic, 2009; Dozier et al., 2017). Many of our participants felt the podcasts were entertaining as one participant describes here:

But Penny Lancaster, Rod Stewart's wife, she did the funniest bit ...she was describing - because she's quite a normal person - and she was describing how she was cooking fish fingers and chips for the kids. She was just - before she realised what was going on, before she was on HRT - and she just had this absolute menopausal rage moment and threw the fish fingers across the kitchen

In addition, participants described the accessible nature of the podcasts, the sense of intimacy, and the role of storytelling as being important features. The accessibility of podcasts means that they can be accessed in transit (Weiner, 2014). In our own study, participants reflected on being more likely to be completing housework, driving, or commuting to work whilst listening to podcasts, as the quotes below illustrate:

Podcasts are the easiest to fit into your life because you can do it as you're either driving or in the house pottering, so it's an easy thing to fit in

When you are walking the dogs, you can do it with your ears. You can be hoovering; you can do so much, and you don't have to stop. We all have busy lives, and I think that is the beauty of podcasts, you can do them while you're doing other things

For those familiar with podcasts, finding relevant series and episodes was straightforward, with participants using their preferred platforms, as one participant explains below:

Very straightforward, I just searched on Spotify, a platform I use a lot

Women who had not used podcasts before found it a little more difficult and did not always enjoy the benefits of listening on the move, for example, if they had accessed the podcasts via their laptop.

> *It could be that as I was accessing on my laptop I was stationery—if I was walking or on a bus using a mobile or similar the experience would have been different?*

> *I guess navigating to try and… I was a bit overwhelmed by the lack of sorting or whatever algorithm Google does for me to make things easier to search for on Spotify and BBC. That was the main challenge*

The tone of voice of the podcast speaker was key in communicating the authenticity of their stories, from their pace, inflections, and emotions. A qualitative study of successful journalism podcasts revealed they used a personal narrative style to foster a sense of intimacy and emotional engagement amongst listeners (Lindgren, 2023). This sense of intimacy was reflected by our own participants:

> *I think the intimacy of a voice, if you're wearing headphones in your ears or something there's the confessional kind of element brought in and it does, yeah, it feels really intimate doesn't it as opposed to just reading a story on the page*

The tone and style of the podcast are important in helping listeners to feel like they are part of the conversation and connect with the host (s) (Heshmat et al., 2018; Perks et al., 2019). Schlütz and Hedder (2022) found that podcast listeners form stronger parasocial relationships with their favourite podcast host when the host shows an interest in listeners, shares personal information, and is seen as more competent, authentic, and unpredictable.

> *And you could almost hear that authenticity I suppose in her voice and that was the best one, it was really good*

Typically, menopause podcasts include an element of experience sharing in which women share stories of their own menopause. This allows listeners to learn about the podcast host or guest as individuals; their openness helps the listeners relate to the speakers and connect to the information which they find informative (Shaw et al., 2022). The storytelling style of podcasts is important in providing an engaging experience (Allen, 2019) but also adds credibility and authenticity to health messages (Kreuter et al., 2007). When an individual hears another person's story, it contributes to their knowledge and understanding of the world (Fisher, 2021). Narrative-based information is more engaging to participants and facilitates positive attitudes, increased knowledge, and greater behavioural intent for changing health behaviours (e.g. Kim et al., 2012; Murphy et al., 2013). Narrative information attracts individuals' attention, is more easily processed, and more accurately retrieved, compared to didactic information (Shaffer et al., 2018).

In their work on menopause podcasts, Shaw et al. (2022) reflect on the importance of supplementing stories or personal narratives with a medical perspective. Positioning health information in the form of narratives may influence patient choice and distract from medical information (Jaramillo et al., 2019; Ubel et al., 2001); however, presenting menopause narratives in podcasts mediated by a healthcare professional or expert can ensure evidence-based information is still presented (Sillence et al., 2026; Shaw et al., 2022).

The podcasts I found they had proper medical people on, that was quite nice, who gave you some really good, balances views

Really interesting, and I've already sent two of the episodes that I listened to a friend. All of them followed the same format and had Q&A sessions with the podcast host, a guest, and a GP

Whilst it can be difficult to evaluate information on menopause (Lopez Burst et al. 2024), some participants described how podcasts took the effort out of finding information.

Probably one of the things about podcasts as well is that you're kind of allowing people's expertise to filter the internet for you. And you can just sit back and be educated passively, you don't have to do any of that searching

Overall, the audible format of the podcasts "made it more human". Podcast listeners feel less alone in their experiences and feel more empowered to make changes in their own lives (Edwards et al., 2021).

> *On the whole I think what I took from it mostly was a sense of empowerment mostly of like, 'okay, you asked, there is a real thing happening to you, it's happening to all these other women too, do something about it, you can go and do something about it*

However, podcasts were not for everyone. A small minority of our study participants preferred the written word or simply found it a difficult medium through which to remember some of the finer details.

> *I didn't really engage with the medium of spoken word. I found it a bit monotonous to be honest and disengaged now and again. I felt some of the information was common sense. I still prefer the written word*

> *There were a few that were too complicated to listen to whilst walking—felt like I needed a paper and pen and a few Google searches to follow the narrative*

Finally, some menopause podcasts have sponsors and those that are linked to pharmaceutical companies are viewed more negatively, and this can be a barrier to engagement (Shaw et al., 2022). Our participants noted similar issues and did not enjoy the adverts within the podcasts.

> *I enjoyed taking time out to sit back and relax on my chair at my desk to listen to the podcast episodes. The only thing I may have got agitated with was the promotion of products within certain episodes*

> *I felt the presenters were a bit false in a way and certainly driven by sponsors—advert breaks were annoying*

Overall, participants found podcasts engaging and informative despite little previous experience with the format. As one participant summed up her experience:

This is a quick, accessible, conversational, private way to learn about a difficult, personal subject that can be done for free (if you already have access to phone/computer/internet), easier than visiting the doctors or collecting leaflets and gives lots of real world examples, case studies and further advice

4.4 Summary

Podcasts appear to be a useful digital health technology for women seeking information about menopause. The array of menopause-related podcast series and individual episodes provides women with the choice to listen to basic information about symptoms and treatments through specific topics that are pertinent to their lives and experiences. Whilst knowing what to search for and choosing appropriate search terms takes time compared with web-based information, the episode titles often provide a way for women to recognise rather than recall topics of interest. The combined format of HCP/expert plus personal experience proved an acceptable balance for our participants and gives reassurance around the credibility of the information, combined with the intimacy and connection of personal narratives.

References

Allen, J. L. (2019). Teaching with narrative nonfiction podcasts. *Journal of Educational Multimedia and Hypermedia, 28*(2), 139–164.

Armstrong, A. W., Idriss, N. Z., & Kim, R. H. (2011). Effects of video-based, online education on behavioral and knowledge outcomes in sunscreen use: A randomized controlled trial. *Patient Education and Counseling, 83*(2), 273–277.

Busselle, R., & Bilandzic, H. (2009). Measuring narrative engagement. *Media Psychology, 12*(4), 321–347.

Dmytryshyn, J., & Selk, A. (2022). Learning on the go: Assessing knowledge gained from medical podcasts created for vulvovaginal disease education. *Journal of Lower Genital Tract Disease, 26*(2), 164–168.

Dozier, D. M., Beach, W. A., Gutzmer, K., & Yagade, A. (2017). The transformative power of authentic conversations about cancer. *Health Communication, 32*(11), 1350–1357.

Edwards, A. L., Shaw, P. A., Halton, C. C., Bailey, S. C., Wolf, M. S., Andrews, E. N., & Cartwright, T. (2021). "It just makes me feel a little less alone": A qualitative exploration of the podcast menopause: Unmuted on women's perceptions of menopause. *Menopause, 28*(12), 1374–1384.

Elilnesan, J., Swaminathan, K., Kumar, V. V., Rajan, V. P., Curran, A., & Rayan, F. (2025). 'Tuning into learning': A scoping review of podcasts and webinars in orthopaedic education. *Journal of Clinical Orthopaedics and Trauma*, Article, 103216.

Sillence, E., Osborne, A. K., Kemp, E., & McKellar, K. (2025). Menopause apps: Personal health tracking, empowerment and epistemic injustice. *Digital Health, 11,* Article 20552076251330782.

Elizabeth, Sillence Alison K., Osborne Caroline, Claisse Abigail C., Durrant (2026). Understanding the challenges of using digital health technologies for menopause information. *Patient Education and Counseling* 142109375-https://doi.org/10.1016/j.pec.2025.109375

Fisher, W. R. (2021). *Human communication as narration: Toward a philosophy of reason, value, and action.* University of South Carolina Press.

Harper, J. C., Phillips, S., Biswakarma, R., Yasmin, E., Saridogan, E., Radhakrishnan, S., & Talaulikar, V. (2022). An online survey of perimenopausal women to determine their attitudes and knowledge of the menopause. *Women's Health, 18,* 17455057221106890.

Harter, L. M. (2019). Storytelling in acoustic spaces: Podcasting as embodied and engaged scholarship. *Health Communication, 34*(1), 125–129.

Heshmat, Y., Yang, L., & Neustaedter, C. (2018). Quality 'alone' time through conversations and storytelling: Podcast listening behaviors and routines. *Graphics Interface.*

Jaramillo, S., Horne, Z., & Goldwater, M. (2019). The impact of anecdotal information on medical decision-making.

Kelly, J. M., Perseghin, A., Dow, A. W., Trivedi, S. P., Rodman, A., & Berk, J. (2022). Learning through listening: A scoping review of podcast use in medical education. *Academic Medicine, 97*(7), 1079–1085.

Kim, H. S., Bigman, C. A., Leader, A. E., Lerman, C., & Cappella, J. N. (2012). Narrative health communication and behavior change: The influence of exemplars in the news on intention to quit smoking. *Journal of Communication, 62*(3), 473–492.

Krawczyk, A., Lau, E., Perez, S., Delisle, V., Amsel, R., & Rosberger, Z. (2012). How to inform: Comparing written and video education interventions to increase human papillomavirus knowledge and vaccination intentions in young adults. *Journal of American College Health, 60*(4), 316–322.

Kreuter, M. W., Green, M. C., Cappella, J. N., Slater, M. D., Wise, M. E., Storey, D., Clark, E. M., O'Keefe, D. J., Erwin, D. O., & Holmes, K. (2007). Narrative communication in cancer prevention and control: A framework to guide research and application. *Annals of Behavioral Medicine, 33*, 221–235.

LaBrosse, L., & Albrecht, J. A. (2013). Pilot intervention with adolescents to increase knowledge and consumption of folate-rich foods based on the health belief model. *International Journal of Consumer Studies, 37*(3), 271–278.

Lindgren, M. (2023). Intimacy and emotions in podcast journalism: A study of award-winning Australian and British podcasts. *Journalism Practice, 17*(4), 704–719.

Lopez Burst, E., Ciolfi Felice, M., & O'Kane, A. A. (2024, May). *Using and appropriating technology to support the menopause journey in the UK*. Proceedings of the CHI Conference on Human Factors in Computing Systems (pp. 1–14).

Militello, L., Sezgin, E., Huang, Y., & Lin, S. (2021). Delivering perinatal health information via a voice interactive app (SMILE): Mixed methods feasibility study. *JMIR Formative Research, 5*(3), e18240.

Murphy, S. T., Frank, L. B., Chatterjee, J. S., & Baezconde-Garbanati, L. (2013). Narrative versus nonnarrative: The role of identification, transportation, and emotion in reducing health disparities. *Journal of Communication, 63*(1), 116–137.

Ofcom. (2024). *Media nations 2024: UK*. https://www.ofcom.org.uk/siteassets/resources/documents/research-and-data/multi-sector/media-nations/2024/media-nations-2024-uk.pdf?v=371192

Osborne, A. K., & Sillence, E. (2025). Accessing information on menopause transition and the role of digital health technologies: A narrative review. *Women & Health*, 1–14.

Perks, L. G., Turner, J. S., & Tollison, A. C. (2019). Podcast uses and gratifications scale development. *Journal of Broadcasting & Electronic Media, 63*(4), 617–634.

Robins, B., Delaney, T., Maher, C., & Singh, B. (2024). Podcasts as a tool for promoting health-related behaviours: A scoping review. *Digital Health, 10*, 20552076241288630.

Robinson, S., & Ritzko, J. (2009). *Podcasts in education: What, why and how?* Allied Academies International Conference. Academy of Educational Leadership. Proceedings.

Ross, L., Ashford, A. D., Bleechington, S. J., Dark, T., & Erwin, D. O. (2010). Applicability of a video intervention to increase informed decision making for prostate-specific antigen testing. *Journal of the National Medical Association, 102*(3), 228–236.

Schlütz, D., & Hedder, I. (2022). Aural parasocial relations: Host–listener relationships in podcasts. *Journal of Radio & Audio Media, 29*(2), 457–474.

Shaffer, V. A., Focella, E. S., Hathaway, A., Scherer, L. D., & Zikmund-Fisher, B. J. (2018). On the usefulness of narratives: An interdisciplinary review and theoretical model. *Annals of Behavioral Medicine, 52*(5), 429–442.

Shaw, P. A., Sumner, A. L., Halton, C. C., Bailey, S. C., Wolf, M. S., Andrews, E. N., & Cartwright, T. (2022). "You're more engaged when you're listening to somebody tell their story": A qualitative exploration into the mechanisms of the podcast 'menopause: Unmuted' for communicating health information. *Patient Education and Counseling, 105*(12), 3494–3500.

Tobin, S. J., & Guadagno, R. E. (2022). Why people listen: Motivations and outcomes of podcast listening. *PLoS One, 17*(4), e0265806.

Turner-McGrievy, G., Kalyanaraman, S., & Campbell, M. K. (2013). Delivering health information via podcast or web: Media effects on psychosocial and physiological responses. *Health Communication, 28*(2), 101–109.

Ubel, P. A., Jepson, C., & Baron, J. (2001). The inclusion of patient testimonials in decision aids: Effects on treatment choices. *Medical Decision Making, 21*(1), 60–68.

Verdusco, L. M. (2016). What are podcasts? *Home Healthcare Now, 34*(4), 224–225.

Weiner, J. (2014). *The voices: Toward a critical theory of podcasting*. https://www.slate.com/articles/arts/ten_years_in_your_ears/2014/12/what_makes_podcasts_so_addictive_and_pleasurable.html

5

Social Media and Menopause Influencers

Abstract In recent years, the number of menopause experts and influencers has increased dramatically. Menopause influencers can encompass medical professionals, people with lived experience, lifestyle coaches, and celebrities. They can focus on specific elements of menopause such as lifestyle, diet and exercise, hormone replacement therapy (HRT) or can focus on specific settings or groups of people, e.g. workplace settings or teachers. Their background, credentials, stated motivations and the information, advice, and services they offer vary considerably. In this chapter, we will (1) introduce the relationship between social media and menopause, (2) provide an overview of menopause influencers in this space, and (3) provide details from our work on women's experiences of using social media for menopause and highlight key findings with relation to social media and menopause narratives.

Keywords Social media · Menopause influencers · Misinformation · Narrative framing · Source credibility

E. Sillence and A. Osborne, *Digital Health Technologies and the Menopause*, Palgrave Studies in Cyberpsychology, https://doi.org/10.1007/978-3-032-25909-7_5

5.1 Social Media and Menopause

The relationship between social media and menopause is one that has come under scrutiny in recent years. The founder of Menopause Cafe, Rachel Weiss, captured the pros and cons for the public in terms of social media and the menopause focusing on its potential for community building and peer connection—a theme we return to in Chapter 6—and importantly on its potential for education (Weiss, 2023). Social media, argues Weiss, provides a quick, accessible way of conveying menopause information in a format that is easily digestible.

However, she also warns that social media often amplifies the negative aspects of menopause, since those suffering "severe symptoms are more likely to search for answers and vent their frustrations" (Weiss, 2023, p. 67). Weiss also highlights the dangers of misinformation around menopause on social media. She argues this can be unintentional or for commercial gain and highlights the volume of social media posts relating to menopause that are advertising services or products (Arseneau et al., 2021). Mansour et al. (2024) have investigated the shift in the perspectives of women and HCPs towards HRT since 2015 and identified media influence, including social media, as one of the key driving factors. They highlight a number of unrealistic expectations they say are created by social media, including the promotion of testosterone to treat low sexual desire, which has led to long waiting lists to see specialist testosterone prescribers.

Social media influencers can reach vast numbers of subscribers and build relationships with them through their social interactions (Senft, 2008). Health influencers focus on health-related topics, sharing information and opinions with their subscribers. Some influencers do not have any professional credentials but focus on sharing personal experiences with subscribers whilst other influencers are experts (such as doctors, nutritionists, and fitness coaches) sharing their knowledge and expertise through social media.

5.2 Menopause Influencers

Menopause influencers encompass everyone from gynaecologists and GPs to lifestyle coaches, nutrition experts, celebrities, and personal experience vloggers. Their backgrounds and credentials may be medical, holistic, experts by experience, or may be unclear. Their area of 'expertise' may be HRT, diet and exercise, lifestyle changes, or setting focused, e.g. workplace-based. Table 5.1 provides examples of menopause influencers with a strong presence on social media. It includes health professionals, media personalities, and coaches. Influencers vary in terms of their specific aim or focus, the number of followers they have, and the extent to which they engage with other media platforms and dissemination avenues. The influencers in Table 5.1 have established careers and or professional credentials, but we know that many influencers rely on sharing personal experiences and establishing a sense of intimacy and connection with followers. These influencers may well focus on different menopause topics and products to those discussed by medical professionals on social media and rely on blending information with subjective viewpoints to engage viewers (Van Poucke, 2025).

5.3 Menopause Information on Social Media

The accessibility of menopause information on social media raises issues around narrative framing and the problem of misinformation. We consider misinformation first before describing a study looking at narrative framing and women's experience of using social media for menopause information.

5.3.1 Misinformation

Misinformation is commonplace within women's health. Arena et al. (2022), for example, report that 75% of women in their study had

Table 5.1 Menopause influencers with a social media presence

Menopause influencer	'Type' of influencer	Description of activity
Dr Louise Newson	Medical doctor and menopause specialist (735 K followers on Instagram).	Provides information on menopause through her website, Instagram, podcasts, and balance app. Runs a menopause clinic. Authored books on menopause, gives talks, and contributes to television programmes answering questions on menopause and hormones.
Davina McCall	Television presenter, menopausal campaigner (2.1 M followers on Instagram).	Presented two menopause TV programmes leading to the so-called Davina effect, shares personal experiences of menopause and HRT. Co-authored book on menopause.
Dr Nighat Arif	GP specialising in women's health, family planning, and menopause care (238 K followers on Instagram).	Posts short menopause information TikTok videos set to lively music often in Urdu and Punjabi, aims to raise awareness on menopause in black and Asian women. Regular contributor to UK television programmes.
Fiona McKay	Menopause career coach (2153 K followers on Instagram).	Founded the menopause maze, providing support and resources for female leaders in terms of their careers and their companies.

encountered online misinformation regarding endometriosis. Reproductive health misinformation is diverse and represents a range of ideological standpoints (Malki et al., 2023). Misleading information can include subtle manipulation and exaggerations, and John et al. (2025) found that 23% of misleading content made medical recommendations that do not align with professional guidelines. In terms of challenging misinformation, women draw on existing knowledge and experience to help fact-check online information; they look at the comments in response to social media posts and check the sentiment of the engagement metrics (Malki et al., 2024).

The literature on social media and menopause specifically suggests a similar issue of misinformation. Whilst 38% of women have used a social media platform for information on nutrition during menopause, half do not find it reliable (Davies & Halliday, 2025) and social media content around hormone treatment for menopause often contains misleading terminology and highlights unregulated products (Gunter, 2022).

5.3.2 The Narrative Framing of Menopause Information on Social Media

The narrative framing of menopause by influencers has led in some cases to tangible, behavioural outcomes. Although on the television rather than on social media, Davina McCall's programmes about menopause (Channel 4, 2021), highlighting personal positive experiences of using HRT, led to some menopause organisations being overwhelmed with requests for information and support and HRT requests going up (see Mansour et al., 2024; Orgad & Rottenberg, 2024). Celebrities like Davina McCall and others have a large social media presence, and this provides a platform for discussing menopause. We know that social media influencers can have positive and negative impacts on health (Powell & Pring, 2024), and whilst 18–22-year-olds believe that their parents' generation are unlikely to get their health information from social media influencers (Pfender & Bleakley, 2024), we know little about what mid-life women themselves think about social media and the menopause narratives they encounter.

5.4 Accessing Menopause Information through Social Media

To understand more about women's experiences with social media for menopause information, we ran a small-scale interview study with a think-aloud element to capture women's engagement with different social media narratives.

Six women who identified as going through the menopause came into the lab to take part in a study about social media and menopause information. During the hour-long individual interviews, we asked women about their experience of and engagement with social media for accessing information on menopause and showed them some social media posts on menopause.

First, we asked our participants to tell us how they had engaged with social media for menopause information so far. We asked them to consider which platforms they had used, whether there were any particular people they followed on social media, and how they considered information across social media in relation to other information sources.

We then showed our participants some screenshots of social media posts that we had taken on World Menopause Day 2024. These 12 posts were taken from Twitter, Facebook, and Instagram and were posted by a range of authors including medical experts, menopause advocates, health organisations, and nutritionists. Before the study, we piloted the posts and sorted them into groups that were representative of de Salis et al's (2018) three interdependent narratives (1) Normality—menopause as a normal, biological process distinct from self, identity, and social transitions; (2) Distress—menopause as a struggle, provoking and expressing distress, and a time of identity loss and social upheaval; and (3) Transformation—menopause as a time of liberation and transformation. Example texts from the social media posts are shown in Table 5.2.

Table 5.2 Example of the messages within the different social media posts and their relevant narrative

Normality	Menopause is a natural stage of a woman's life when monthly menstruation also known as periods ends.
	Menopause is a natural part of life, not a cause for embarrassment or shame.
Distress	Symptoms of menopause often last for many years or decades. Low hormones last forever.
	We need to stop labelling the menopause as a natural process ...we should be calling it what it is: a long-term hormone deficiency.
Transformation	Menopause is an incredible phase, full of change, challenges, and growth.
	Menopause can kick us into our powerful next chapter.

We were interested in what our participants thought about these posts, their messaging, and the source. We asked participants to think aloud whilst looking at the posts. This involved trying to tell us everything they were thinking whilst reading the posts, whether this be about the message itself, how it made them feel, or what they would take away from the post.

5.4.1 Current Experiences With Social Media for Menopause

Our participants had relatively limited experience with social media for menopause. One participant talked about using Facebook groups in the past, and only one participant described their current use of Instagram for menopause information.

> *I engage fairly regularly. Eve appeal as well. Their social media presence is really good. I know that's not necessarily a menopause related charity, but sometimes they do have menopause content on there and so I follow them. And I follow a couple of female menopause specialists on Instagram as well*

Other participants had social media accounts often set up by their children, but did not engage with social media for menopause information.

> *My daughter made me an Instagram account. She made me a Tiktok account. She sends me things on there, you know, but they're just funny videos or funny memes or things like that. Which kind of a month goes past when she goes. have you seen that? I sent you this and I'm like, no, I don't go on it*

Social media was not usually the first place our participants went to for health-related information, but they thought that it could be a useful way of increasing general awareness of health information rather than for finding an answer to a specific question.

> *Yeah, I do it more and more frequently, I guess. Yeah. My dad is suffering COPD and I'm just going to ask Insta as well, try and get a more general*

knowledge about COPD. From insta. But I don't see it as a source of facts. I think I just increase in my general knowledge (by using it)

As with online groups and peer support (see Chapter 6), there was a sense for some participants that social media might become more useful and relevant in the future as their needs increased.

I'll probably need it. Yeah. So it's not I feel I'm not in that need now, but I guess I'm on Facebook, I use that or I could use that should I need do

5.4.2 Evaluating Social Media Posts on Menopause

Message: Whilst women differed in their preference for HRT versus alternative treatments, there was broad agreement across the interviews that a more positive perspective or narrative was preferential over a negative '*doom and gloom*' message. That said, it was important to find the right balance. For some women, they rejected the overtly negative talk that focused solely on problems, yet they also rejected an overly upbeat approach in which messages discussed embracing and even celebrating menopause. For some people, this was simply too emotion-laden, but for others, those messages did not fit with their own experience, and they found it '*belittling*'. Once again, we saw that the narrative of the social media posts needed to match the participant's perspective or outlook on menopause. With participants saying, "*we look for what we need to know*" *and "that really speaks to me"*.

Language: Participants commented on the specific language used in the social media posts. Depending on people's perspectives, certain words were comforting or disempowering, for example, 'condition' was helpful for a participant who had experienced early menopause but another said "*I don't want to see it as a condition*" and *"I don't want to hear 'forever' that's not nice"*. Similarly, words such as 'growth', 'sisterhood', and 'community' were both appealing and off-putting to different women. Again, this reflected women's individual perspectives on menopause. "*I have problems with language like that because of my own experience*".

Tone: All our participants picked up on the tone of the messages, describing many as 'calm', 'kindly', 'friendly', 'nice', and 'gentle'. Others were described as 'boring', 'angry', and for several women, a 'cringey feel' to the messages signalled a rejection of the social media post.

In a recent follow-on survey study, we found that how menopause is framed on social media can meaningfully influence women's immediate affective responses to online information. We showed women posts from one of the narratives from the study described above (distressing, normal, and transformative). We found that framing social media posts about menopause in distressing terms increased negative emotional responses such as worry. We also found that both distressing and transformative posts were seen as less representative of health professionals compared to normal posts, and transformative posts were also seen as less representative of newspapers or TV.

5.5 Discussion

More work needs to be done to understand the role of social media in menopause information and support. In our very small-scale study, participants were familiar with some menopause influencers but less familiar with their social presence. The more recognisable influencers had a presence across multiple platforms including television and print media. Our participants, although relatively light users of social media, focused less on the source of the social media posts and more on the message itself, noting the positive or negative narrative, the language, and tone of the message.

Many participants did not feel they were learning anything new from this format, but agreed that social media information raised general awareness about menopause. The narrative or 'feel' of the post was important, and that is what our participants responded to. As an accessible and potentially influential source of information about menopause, the way social media posts are framed is important. In our studies, women either favoured balanced or normal narratives over transformative or distressing narratives. Putting aside source credibility, positively framed messages are more effective than those with a negative frame in terms of attitudes and behavioural intentions across other contexts (Kim & Kim, 2014), but we also know that there are well-documented negativity effects, where people often treat negative information as more informative and remember it more strongly (Baumeister et al., 2001; Kensinger, 2009). Negative language often travels better on social media platforms (Brady et al., 2017), and recent qualitative research on peri/menopause messages received as anticipatory education found that participants tended to judge memorable messages as negative or ambivalent, suggesting cognitive biases favouring negative menopause information (Rubinsky et al., 2025).

Finally, to return to influencers, source credibility is important in health communication. Whilst credibility used to be driven by expertise, where expertise referred to medical credentials, the advent of social media has meant that the experiential expert is also a considered form of source credibility (Hocevar et al., 2017). Lived experience provides a compelling form of communication with personal narratives seen as more engaging and transportive (Green & Brock, 2000). Morris (2021) has argued that the way celebrities, for example, communicate about menopause by combining their personal experience with other forms of expert input may be a more effective way of engaging with women about menopause.

References

Arena, A., Degli Esposti, E., Orsini, B., Verrelli, L., Rodondi, G., Lenzi, J., et al. (2022). The social media effect: The impact of fake news on women affected by endometriosis. A prospective observational study. *European Journal of Obstetrics & Gynecology and Reproductive Biology, 274*, 101–105.

Arseneau, M. E., Backonja, U., Litchman, M. L., Karimanfard, R., Sheng, X., & Taylor-Swanson, L. (2021). #Menopause on instagram: A mixed-methods study. *Menopause, 28*(4), 391–399.

Baumeister, R. F., Bratslavsky, E., Finkenauer, C., & Vohs, K. D. (2001). Bad is stronger than good. *Review of General Psychology, 5*(4), 323–370.

Brady, W. J., Wills, J. A., Jost, J. T., Tucker, J. A., & Van Bavel, J. J. (2017). Emotion shapes the diffusion of moralized content in social networks. *Proceedings of the National Academy of Sciences, 114*(28), 7313–7318.

Channel 4. (2021). *Davina McCall: Sex, myths and the menopause*. https://www.channel4.com/programmes/davina-mccall-sex-myths-and-the-menopause

Davies, E., & Halliday, V. (2025). Nutrition information and the menopause: An online survey of perimenopausal and menopausal women. *Post Reproductive Health, 31*(2), 65–72.

Green, M. C., & Brock, T. C. (2000). The role of transportation in the persuasiveness of public narratives. *Journal of Personality and Social Psychology, 79*(5), 701–721.

Gunter, J. (2022). Addressing the challenges of online misinformation and unregulated products in the clinical management of menopause. *Obstetrics & Gynecology*, 10–1097.

Hocevar, K. P., Metzger, M., & Flanagin, A. J. (2017). Source credibility, expertise, and trust in health and risk messaging. In *Oxford Research Encyclopedia of Communication*.

John, J. N., Gorman, S., Scales, D., & Gorman, J. (2025). Online misleading information about women's reproductive health: A narrative review. *Journal of General Internal Medicine, 40*(5), 1123–1131.

Kensinger, E. A. (2009). Remembering the details: Effects of emotion. *Emotion Review, 1*(2), 99–113.

Kim, S.-B., & Kim, D.-Y. (2014). The effects of message framing and source credibility on green messages in hotels. *Cornell Hospitality Quarterly, 55*(1), 64–75.

Malki, L. M., Patel, D., & Singh, A. (2023, August). *A mixed-methods analysis of women's health misinformation on social media*. IFIP Conference on Human-Computer Interaction (pp. 419–428). Springer Nature.

Malki, L. M., Patel, D., & Singh, A. (2024). "The headline was so wild that I had to check": An exploration of women's encounters with health misinformation on social media. Proceedings of the ACM on Human-Computer Interaction, 8(CSCW1), 1–26.

Mansour, D., Barber, K., Chalk, G., Noble, N., Digpal, A. A. S., Talaulikar, V., & Gray, S. (2024). The evolving perspective of menopause management in the United Kingdom. Women's Health, 20, Article 17455057241288641.

Morris, E. (2021). Learning from celebrities and influencers—The future of menopause communication? *Post Reproductive Health, 27*(3), 131–132.

Orgad, S., & Rottenberg, C. (2024). The menopause moment: The rising visibility of 'the change' in UK news coverage. *European Journal of Cultural Studies, 27*(4), 519–539.
Pfender, E., & Bleakley, A. (2024). An elicitation study to understand young adults' beliefs about seeking health information from social media influencers. *Qualitative Health Research, 34*(3), 205–216.
Powell, J., & Pring, T. (2024). The impact of social media influencers on health outcomes: Systematic review. *Social Science & Medicine, 340*, 116472.
Rubinsky, V., Tolman, C., & Cooke-Jackson, A. (2025). "just deal with it": Memorable messages about menopause as anticipatory education. *American Journal of Sexuality Education*, 1–26.
Senft, T. M. (2008). *Camgirls: Celebrity & community in the age of social networks*. Peter Lang.
Van Poucke, M. (2025). Negotiating the maze of menopause misinformation: A comparative analysis of stance in health influencer versus medical professional discourse. *Atlantic Journal of Communication*, 1–23.
Weiss, R. (2023). Menopause and social media: Pros and cons for the general public. *Maturitas, 174*, 67–68.

6

Peer Support and Menopause

Abstract Peer support has been shown to be an important resource for many health conditions, especially those that are chronic, less common, or those that are potentially stigmatiszed (Ziebland & Wyke, 2012; Coulson et al., 2007). Whilst many women receive their menopause information from friends and family, not everyone has these connections, and some women want to explore different spaces for discussing menopause or importantly be able to seek out different experiences of menopause. This chapter explores the role of peer support in menopause and is organised as follows: (1) we introduce the notion of peer support in menopause including the importance of friends and family and work colleagues. (2) We describe online peer support and provide an overview of what this looks like and review the literature describing the role of such support networks. Section (3) details findings from studies, including our own research, examining online peer support for menopause, and finally, (4) we highlight ongoing issues for peer support around representation.

Keywords Online peer support · Online health communities · Menopause networks · Normalisation · Anonymity

E. Sillence and A. Osborne, *Digital Health Technologies and the Menopause*, Palgrave Studies in Cyberpsychology, https://doi.org/10.1007/978-3-032-25909-7_6

6.1 Peer Support in Menopause

The way in which messages about reproductive health transitions from menarche to menopause are communicated is important in terms of self-care and wellbeing. We know that positive communication improves wellbeing whilst poor communication leads to increased feelings of shame and increased body dissatisfaction. The messages that are communicated intergenerationally often inform perceptions of menarche or menopause (Field-Springer et al., 2018). Female relatives, particularly mothers, are an important source of information on menstruation and menopause. These connections provide opportunities for meaningful information exchange and support, but can also be unsatisfactory. Menstruation discussions may be limited to a single conversation, can often be restricted to issues of hygiene, and such discussions are rarely revisited or updated. Likewise, adolescent girls receive little or no information about the menopause, and for younger women, their representations of menopause and perimenopause may be limited and medicalised (Hayfield & Campbell, 2022).

Women often turn to their friends for support during menopause (Koch & Mansfield, 2004). A survey of perimenopausal women suggested that 63% of women (Harper et al., 2022) had sought information on menopause from friends, and we know that whilst social support is important for physical and mental health outcomes, insufficient support can leave women feeling isolated during menopause (Koch & Mansfield, 2004). Peer support is also valuable to women in the workplace. Talking to colleagues about shared menopause experiences, symptoms, and management strategies available is highly valued by women. This includes informal chats with colleagues as well as discussions in locally organised menopause cafes (Hobson & Dennis, 2024). Menopause cafes, started by Rachel Weiss, provide spaces for women to share experiences and ask questions. Cafes follow a therapeutic rather than a medical model and empower participants to seek out information for themselves and to make their own decisions based on their own experiences (Weiss, 2020). Beyond in-person peer support, Koch and

Mansfield (2004) suggest that during menopause women may need to develop new social networks including those online in order to access informational and emotional support.

Table 6.1 Different types of peer experiences

Type of peer experience	Example	Description of the resource
Online collections of video and audio experiences	Healthtalk https://healthtalk.org/introduction/menopause/	Text, audio, or video clips of specific aspects of menopause experience—As part of narrative is not interactive
Online groups and forums	Menopause Matters forum Dedicated to menopause topics https://www.menopausematters.co.uk/forum/	Interactive with threading and some organisation and topics, sometimes with user profiles and moderators/admin, sometimes searchable, anonymity varies
Blogs	Menopause blog https://www.hud.ac.uk/news/wellbeing-blogs/nikkis-menopause-blog/ https://www.essex.ac.uk/blog/posts/2024/10/17/menopause-case-study-four	Individual posts, sometimes longer format, sometimes invite comments
Podcasts	Menopause unmuted https://www.pfizer.com/stories/podcasts/menopause	Audio recordings often split into separate episodes discussing different aspects of menopause and menopause experiences. Can be candid and detailed usually informal or conversational style

6.2 Online Peer Experiences and Support

Online peer experiences take a number of different forms. Whilst peer support communities and forums are more common, peer experiences can be embedded within websites, exist as standalone blogs, curated content, or as podcasts (see Table 6.1 for menopause-specific examples). Peer experiences, despite varying in terms of their interactivity, have the power to resonate with individuals, increasing emotional connection and reducing feelings of being alone (Edwards et al., 2021).

Most peer experiences arguably sit within online health communities (OHCs). These provide a space for people to engage with others experiencing similar health conditions and challenges, and typically provide anonymous access to members 24 hours a day. The majority of studies examining peer support have focused on OHCs to understand their role in providing support to individuals across a number of different health conditions.

Online health communities provide a place for people to exchange information, support, and experiential advice. OHCs exist for a large variety of health and wellbeing conditions, including those that are rarer, less well understood, or potentially stigmatising and have been studied in relation to a wide range of health issues including people living with dementia (Talbot & Coulson, 2023), paediatric stroke survivors and their families (Wright et al., 2024), HIV/AIDS (Mo & Coulson, 2013), diabetes (Brady et al., 2017), infertility (O'Connell et al., 2021), and PCOS (Holbrey & Coulson, 2013).

Much of the literature has focused on the types of information and support exchanged within these communities focusing on informational and social support in particular (Coulson, 2005; Coulson et al., 2007; Holbrey & Coulson, 2013; Smedley et al., 2015). Others have examined the affordances (Shoebotham & Coulson, 2016; Yeshua-Katz, 2021), advice exchange processes (Sillence, 2013), or the role of specific user groups such as moderators or administrators (Coulson & Shaw, 2013; Smedley & Coulson, 2017) or superusers—those users contributing the majority of content to OHCs (De Simoni et al., 2020).

Researchers have also noted the importance of the health condition and the underlying ethos of the community to the type of support that is exchanged (Mo et al., 2009; Sillence et al., 2013).

Other studies have focused on the motivations for engaging with OHCs or the potential impact of engaging with OHCs. For example, Coulson (2013) found that the main reasons for accessing an OHC were to find others in a similar situation, to learn new information about the condition, or to share experiences. Mo and Coulson (2011) have argued that participation in OHCs promotes patient empowerment through four activities, receiving useful information, receiving social support, finding positive meaning, and helping others. Sillence and Bussey (2017) have examined the role of OHC in decision-making, noting that OHCs prompt decision-making as well as allowing people to evaluate and confirm decisions they have already made. Ziebland & Wyke (2012) suggest that online peer experiences can feed into seven activities: (1) Finding information, (2) Feeling supported, (3) Maintaining relationships with others, (4) Experiencing health services, (5) Learning to relate the story, (6) visualising disease, and (7) Affecting behaviour. Finally, Sillence et al. (2014) have used an engagement framework to help explain why people engage with some peer support experiences and not others. They describe four processes critical to meaningful engagement with peer experiences. Individuals assess who is making the contribution and what they are saying. Here, participants look at factors such as the age and gender of the author, their location, and circumstances. They also scrutinise what is being said and ask themselves, for example, whether it is a request for information, a message of support, advice, or venting. They then compare online stories with their own experiences, in part to see how relevant the experience is for them, was it an appropriate, useful, or resonant experience, and finally to assess the extent to which they could add their own stories.

The anonymity afforded by many online health communities is an important factor for people accessing peer support. Stigma emphasises the importance of anonymity (Rains, 2018) although many newer-generation online peer communities result in high levels of visibility (Yeshua-Katz, 2021). For OHCs where discussion spaces are underpinned by other platforms such as Facebook or WhatsApp, some of these issues have become more complex. In these cases, anonymity is not guaranteed or may not be desired. WhatsApp groups, for example, may develop around informal friendship groups that also chat about health topics such as menopause or are more formalised support groups that people join based around a local area or health centre or around a health topic, e.g. pregnancy and parenting (Yadav et al., 2022) or endometriosis (Wilson et al., 2022). Platforms may afford different levels of visibility and suggest a safer space for support (Yeshua-Katz, 2021). Individuals may also be mindful of sharing phone numbers and having private content screenshotted and shared (Yadav et al., 2022). Individuals may be sensitive to the different privacy affordances of platforms and use this in making decisions about which platforms to use and their disclosure preferences (O'Leary et al., 2020).

6.3 Online Peer Support and Menopause

Despite the reported benefits of engaging with online peer support reported in Section 6.2, there are relatively few studies focusing on how individuals use online peer support for menopause. We know that women report using the internet and social media for online information (Aljumah et al., 2023; Harper et al., 2022), but what about online peer support?

Back in 2007, Sillence et al. (2007) published a study looking at how individuals trust online health information. The study focused on women experiencing menopause who were deciding whether or not to take HRT. The findings showed that women sought out and valued content that was written by people similar to themselves. Information that was clearly relevant to their experience was preferred, and women were drawn to personal stories that appeared on websites or on forums.

More recently, Lazar et al. (2019) carried out an analysis of messages posted to a subreddit forum. They focused on women's accounts of menopause and presented findings that speak to both menopause experiences specifically and to the value of online peer support more broadly. The study details how women find that medical discourse is insufficient to describe their experiences. The brief, sanitised terminology does not capture the intensity of the physical and mental experiences associated with menopause. Women also capture their negative experiences with medical professionals and use the subreddit forum to push back against ageist and gendered views. The forum provides a safe space for discussing feelings associated with transforming bodies and intimate experiences with partners. The analysis speaks to the fundamentals of online peer support in which women find support in a 'virtual sisterhood', are able to share and read about heterogeneous experiences, and can use the forum as a way of making sense of personal experiences of menopause.

Rushworth and Sillence (2023) aimed to explore the types of messages that people post to online peer support spaces for menopause. They collected data from a public Facebook group on menopause and undertook a thematic analysis of the messages that were posted in response to Davina McCall's TV documentaries on menopause (Channel 4, 2021). As explained in previous chapters, these documentaries saw TV presenter Davina McCall recall her own menopause experience and use of HRT. Rushworth and Sillence (2023) observed that women posting on the Facebook group were very willing to share their own experiences of menopause, disclosing sometimes quite personal information. The content of their posts was captured in six themes:

1. *Raising awareness*—In this theme, posters express a sense of gratitude that Davina McCall is challenging stereotypes and taboos and demystifying menopause. Posters describe the importance of raising the profile of menopause across the general public more broadly. The key thing here is to make it acceptable to talk about menopause.
2. *A lightbulb moment*—This theme captures the way many posters credited the TV programme as the moment they recognised their own menopause experiences. For some people, they only connected the different signs and symptoms to menopause after hearing about other people's experiences in the documentary. Many people referred to this recognition as a sort of 'lightbulb moment'.
3. *This is normal*—Many posters identified not only with Davina McCall but also the other women portrayed in the documentary. Here, posters expressed their realisation that they were 'not alone' and that their symptoms were normal. Women were relieved not to

be 'going mad' and thankful for menopause being normalised in this way.

4. *Taking on the professionals*—This theme captures the increased confidence and empowerment expressed by many posters as they described feeling emboldened to speak to their healthcare professional. For some, this discussion centred on a renewed 'battle for HRT', but for others it represented the start of further research or making the first appointment to find out more.
5. *What about me?* For some posters, the messaging around HRT did not feel inclusive. This theme captures the sense that many people cannot or do not want to take HRT and that approaches to menopause must be holistic and inclusive in nature. Sharing different menopause experiences and seeking alternative approaches was a small but significant part of this online community.
6. *What should I be doing?*—This final theme describes the need for continued information or advice for people going through menopause. For those posters who were well aware of their symptoms and perhaps already taking treatment, many had specific questions regarding their menopause or HRT. Posters sought specific guidance and input from peers via this online group.

Analysing the content of messages posted to online forums and groups provides an insight into how women are sharing information and advice with peers. Peer support allows women to normalise their experiences and understand more about their menopause and how to move forward with treatment options. However, this form of analysis does not help us to understand motivations for sharing, the experience of engaging with peers, or potential limitations with online peer support.

In a series of recent studies (Sillence et al., 2025a, 2025b), a total of 45 women were asked about their use of digital resources for menopause. Some of those women were asked to use online groups and forums for the first time, whilst others commented on their use of such forums for menopause over the years. Using this complementary methodological approach, we were able to explore attitudes towards and experiences of online peer support.

Women in these studies described why it was important to be able to access a different type of information from that found on websites. For example, 'Jackie' had already been using a menopause app to gain a basic understanding of menopause, but decided to join a number of Facebook groups in order to find out what menopause was 'really like'. Jackie thought that online support groups felt 'warmer' than apps or websites, and she felt like she was 'talking at a coffee morning sort of thing'. People in the groups shared tips and information, for example, about supplements. Jackie also described how she could use the groups to ask what might sound like silly questions:

> *Nobody tells you silly things like because the HRT is well it's a plaster basically it leaves like a plaster residue when you take it off just simple things like that, the nurse never mentioned that never mentioned skin irritation and it was only like from these other ladies like on these Facebook pages saying you know what use a little bit of baby oil or use this I've used that try it*

Women felt that the value of online peer support was dependent on where an individual was in their menopause journey. Below, 'Sharon' describes how her engagement with online peer support has changed over the course of her menopause journey.

> *And it's like when I was pulling my hair out and screaming inside... And I was very much into Facebook, so I found groups on Facebook, because I was using Facebook all the time. And I found these groups and everyone was screaming on those groups and that really suited me. And I thought, "This is great." And I did a bit of screaming as well, a little bit here and there. But ever since going into post-menopause, and especially these past couple of years, and especially ever since starting HRT, I've just completely calmed down and I've just not gone back. So, I think it depends where you are in that cycle*

For those women in our study using online forums for the first time (Sillence, Osborne, Claisse, & Durrant, 2025), engagement with peer support was often difficult. Many people struggled to engage with the forums and found the volume of information overwhelming. Navigation within online groups could be daunting with limited search functionality. Posts within a certain thread or subheading did not always stay on topic making conversations difficult to follow and women reported getting lost or being led into random off-topic discussions. They were not always able to find answers to specific questions and found it difficult to reconcile different opinions or contradictory information. It was sometimes challenging for women to imagine how online forums would be a useful information resource.

> *I didn't have any questions to ask and as a total forum novice I didn't feel 'brave' enough to ask or answer any questions. I have never thought to use forums as an information source*

> *I suppose, for me, I just found it a bit overwhelming, the online group. It was just a lot to look through and a lot to, sort of, I guess, find what you were looking for*

Many of our participants expressed a preference for face-to-face support and appreciated having trusted family and friends. Online peers were still an 'unknown quantity', and it was not always clear that their advice could be trusted. However, women did recognise that online forums may provide valuable emotional and social support especially if offline support networks were not available.

> *But that's what I'm saying, either colleagues or friends, because, again, we're going through similar things, so I learn from them, who you can trust. I think for me, it's a trust thing. People online, I don't know who they are*

> *I would feel a bit strange, putting my question to the world, I'd rather find my answer myself. But then, if I needed to or it was appropriate, it felt also.. well for all the people who are throwing everything in, it still felt quite a safe environment, there was not much negativity*

Online groups and forums can be a valuable resource for people going through menopause. They provide a space for conversations that do not or cannot happen elsewhere. This might involve sharing experiences, describing symptoms, and simply venting frustrations. Some people engage actively with these spaces, asking questions and offering responses to posters. For others, simply reading that other women are experiencing similar problems is comforting and online peers are a valuable resource for normalising menopause. For those new to online groups, they can feel overwhelming, and it can be difficult to know how to get started. Finding specific information is not always straightforward, not least because of the structure and organisation of online groups, which often contain multiple threads with topics quickly changing as discussions progress.

6.4 Discussion

Peer support, whether it is in person or online, continues to be an important source of information and support for people going through menopause. In-person support remains pivotal, with friends perceived to be the most important source of support amongst women with menopausal symptoms (Duffy et al., 2012). Partners also remain an important source of support to women during menopause (Cowell et al., 2024), and emotional support from spouses plays a role in mitigating anxiety and depression (Namazi et al., 2019). Participation in offline support groups has positive effects. It can alleviate some of the vasomotor symptoms of menopause and improve quality of life (Yazdkhasti et al., 2012). But women experience barriers to participating in support groups with fears around crying in public and being perceived as attention seeking when discussing symptoms and key concerns (Duffy et al., 2011).

Online health communities have a different role to play in the sense that they can afford anonymity and a safe space to vent frustrations around symptoms, to complain about poor treatment or support from workplaces and from HCPs, and to ask seemingly trivial questions. Unlike offline support groups, participants do not have to fear crying in front of others or posting often-asked questions. Not all online groups are alike, and the tone and style of groups can vary enormously. Some groups focus on emotional support, whereas others are centred on information exchange (Armstrong et al., 2012). This helps the identity of the online support group and in turn its longevity, but it inevitably influences the type of content or direction of topics and conversations (Tang et al., 2021) so that the underlying ethos or narrative of a group varies. Hence, we see online peer support for menopause that focuses on medical treatments or holistic approaches to menopause, and not all menopause narratives are necessarily represented (as highlighted in chapter 5). The value women can glean from participation in online support groups appears to relate to the stage of menopause, the type of information or support required, and of course is affected by personal preference. Like all groups, some voices are louder than others; some narratives are stronger than others. This means that not everyone feels represented within such communities (Lopez Burst et al., 2024). A strong focus on HRT, for example, can feel alienating for women who do not want to or are unable to take hormonal-based treatments. Women may feel that certain voices are foregrounded with poor representation of certain age groups, sexualities, and relationship and caring responsibility statuses.

For our UK participants, voices from the US or Australia were less useful simply based on healthcare system differences and differing treatment names. Here, the issue of whether people can trust information is important. We know that people like but do not necessarily automatically trust peer experiences (Sillence et al., 2013) and seek to corroborate information they find within personal accounts of health and wellbeing (Sillence et al., 2019). Finally, it may be useful to explore further how online peer support may have a role to play in fostering offline connections. Online groups often have a local element with the opportunity to meet up face to face. People value organised peer support although many would still prefer to talk to friends over a cup of tea. They are looking for friends who also discuss menopause rather than a menopause-focused discussion group (Sillence et al., 2025a, 2025b).

References

Aljumah, R., Phillips, S., & Harper, J. C. (2023). An online survey of post-menopausal women to determine their attitudes and knowledge of the menopause. *Post Reproductive Health, 29*(2), 67–84.

Armstrong, N., Koteyko, N., & Powell, J. (2012). 'Oh dear, should I really be saying that on here?': Issues of identity and authority in an online diabetes community. *Health, 16*(4), 347–365.

Brady, E., Segar, J., & Sanders, C. (2017). Accessing support and empowerment online: The experiences of individuals with diabetes. *Health Expectations, 20*(5), 1088–1095.

Channel 4. (2021). *Davina McCall: Sex, myths and the menopause*. https://www.channel4.com/programmes/davina-mccall-sex-myths-and-the-menopause

Coulson, N. S. (2005). Receiving social support online: An analysis of a computer-mediated support group for individuals living with irritable bowel syndrome. *Cyberpsychology & Behavior, 8*(6), 580–584.

Coulson, N. S. (2013). How do online patient support communities affect the experience of inflammatory bowel disease? An online survey. *JRSM Short Reports, 4*(8), 2042533313478004.

Coulson, N. S., Buchanan, H., & Aubeeluck, A. (2007). Social support in cyberspace: A content analysis of communication within a Huntington's disease online support group. *Patient Education and Counseling, 68*(2), 173–178.

Coulson, N. S., & Shaw, R. L. (2013). Nurturing health-related online support groups: Exploring the experiences of patient moderators. *Computers in Human Behavior, 29*(4), 1695–1701.

Cowell, A. C., Gilmour, A., & Atkinson, D. (2024). Support mechanisms for women during menopause: Perspectives from social and professional structures. *Women, 4*(1), 53–72.

De Simoni, A., Shah, A. T., Fulton, O., Parkinson, J., Sheikh, A., Panzarasa, P., Leach, J., & Griffiths, C. J. (2020). Superusers' engagement in asthma online communities: Asynchronous web-based interview study. *Journal of Medical Internet Research, 22*(6), Article e18185.

Duffy, O., Iversen, L., & Hannaford, P. C. (2011). The menopause 'it's somewhere between a taboo and a joke. A focus group study. *Climacteric, 14*(4), 497–505.

Duffy, O. K., Iversen, L., & Hannaford, P. C. (2012). The impact and management of symptoms experienced at midlife: A community-based study of women in Northeast Scotland. *BJOG: An International Journal of Obstetrics & Gynaecology, 119*, 554–564.

Edwards, A. L., Shaw, P. A., Halton, C. C., Bailey, S. C., Wolf, M. S., Andrews, E. N., & Cartwright, T. (2021). "it just makes me feel a little less alone": A qualitative exploration of the podcast menopause: Unmuted on women's perceptions of menopause. *Menopause, 28*(12), 1374–1384.

Field-Springer, K., Randall-Griffiths, D., & Reece, C. (2018). From menarche to menopause: Understanding multigenerational reproductive health milestones. *Health Communication, 33*(6), 733–742.

Harper, J. C., Phillips, S., Biswakarma, R., Yasmin, E., Saridogan, E., Radhakrishnan, S., & Talaulikar, V. (2022). An online survey of perimenopausal women to determine their attitudes and knowledge of the menopause. *Women's Health, 18*, 17455057221106890.

Hayfield, N., & Campbell, C. (2022). Students' representations of menopause and perimenopause: Out of control bodies and empathetic expert doctors. *Sex Roles, 87*(7), 365–378.

Hobson, G., & Dennis, N. (2024). "I can't be dealing with this brain fog": A workplace focus group study investigating factors underpinning the menopausal experience for NHS staff. *Maturitas, 180*.

Holbrey, S., & Coulson, N. S. (2013). A qualitative investigation of the impact of peer to peer online support for women living with polycystic ovary syndrome. *BMC Women's Health, 13*, 1–9.

Koch, P. B., & Mansfield, P. K. (2004). Facing the unknown: Social support during the menopausal transition. *Women and Therapy, 27*(3–4), 179–194.

Lazar, A., Su, N. M., Bardzell, J., & Bardzell, S. (2019, May). Parting the Red Sea: Sociotechnical systems and lived experiences of menopause. *Proceedings of the 2019 CHI Conference on Human Factors in Computing Systems* (pp. 1–16).

Lopez Burst, E., Ciolfi Felice, M., & O'Kane, A. A. (2024, May). Using and appropriating technology to support the menopause journey in the UK. *Proceedings of the CHI Conference on Human Factors in Computing Systems* (pp. 1–14).

Mo, P. K., Malik, S. H., & Coulson, N. S. (2009). Gender differences in computer-mediated communication: A systematic literature review of online health-related support groups. *Patient Education and Counseling, 75*(1), 16–24.

Mo, P. K. H., & Coulson, N. S. (2011). Developing a model for online support group use, empowering processes and psychosocial outcomes for individuals living with HIV/AIDS. *Psychology & Health, 27*(4), 445–459.

Mo, P. K. H., & Coulson, N. S. (2013). Online support group use and psychological health for individuals living with HIV/AIDS. *Patient Education and Counseling, 93*(3), 426–432.

Namazi, M., Sadeghi, R., & Behboodi Moghadam, Z. (2019). Social determinants of health in menopause: An integrative review. *International Journal of Women's Health, 11*, 637–647.

O'Connell, S. B. L., Gelgoot, E. N., Grunberg, P. H., Schinazi, J., Da Costa, D., Dennis, C. L., Genest, D., & Zelkowitz, P. (2021). 'I felt less alone knowing I could contribute to the forum': Psychological distress and use of an online infertility peer support forum. *Health Psychology and Behavioral Medicine, 9*(1), 128–148.

O'Leary, K., Coulson, N., Perez-Vallejos, E., & McAuley, D. (2020). Towards understanding how individuals with inflammatory bowel disease use contemporary social media platforms for health-related discourse. *Computers in Human Behavior, 112*, 106463.

Rushworth, S., & Sillence, E. (2023, July). *The Davina effect: Celebrity disclosures and online discussions of the (peri)menopause*. BPS Cyberpsychology Conference, Newcastle upon Tyne.

Rains, S. A. (2018). *Coping with illness digitally*. The MIT Press.

Shoebotham, A., & Coulson, N. S. (2016). Therapeutic affordances of online support group use in women with endometriosis. *Journal of Medical Internet Research, 18*(5), e109.

Sillence, E. (2013). Giving and receiving peer advice in an online breast cancer support group. *Cyberpsychology, Behavior, and Social Networking, 16*(6), 480–485.

Sillence, E., Blythe, J. M., Briggs, P., & Moss, M. (2019). A revised model of trust in internet-based health information and advice: Cross-sectional questionnaire study. *Journal of Medical Internet Research, 21*(11), e11125.

Sillence, E., Briggs, P., Harris, P. R., & Fishwick, L. (2007). How do patients evaluate and make use of online health information? *Social Science & Medicine, 64*(9), 1853–1862.

Sillence, E., & Bussey, L. (2017). Changing hospitals, choosing chemotherapy and deciding you've made the right choice: Understanding the role of online support groups in different health decision-making activities. *Patient Education and Counseling, 100*(5), 994–999.

Sillence, E., Hardy, C., & Briggs, P. (2013, May). *Why do't we trust health websites that help us help each other? An analysis of online peer-to-peer healthcare*. Proceedings of the 5th Annual ACM Web Science Conference (pp. 396–404).

Sillence, E., Hardy, C., Harris, P. R., & Briggs, P. (2014, April). *Modeling patient engagement in peer-to-peer healthcare*. Proceedings of the 23rd International Conference on World Wide Web (pp. 481–486).

Sillence, E., Osborne, A. K., Claisse, C., & Durrant, A. C. (2025). Understanding the challenges of using digital health technologies for menopause information. *Patient Education and Counseling*, Article 109375.

Sillence, E., Osborne, A. K., Kemp, E., & McKellar, K. (2025). Menopause apps: Personal health tracking, empowerment and epistemic injustice. *Digital. Health, 11*, 20552076251330782.

Smedley, R., Coulson, N., Gavin, J., Rodham, K., & Watts, L. (2015). Online social support for complex regional pain syndrome: A content analysis of support exchanges within a newly launched discussion forum. *Computers in Human Behavior, 51*, 53–63.

Smedley, R. M., & Coulson, N. S. (2017). A thematic analysis of messages posted by moderators within health-related asynchronous online support forums. *Patient Education and Counseling, 100*(9), 1688–1693.

Talbot, C. V., & Coulson, N. S. (2023). 'I found it the only place that spoke the same language': A thematic analysis of messages posted to an online peer support discussion forum for people living with dementia. *Age and Ageing, 52*(1), afac330.

Tang, J., Yao, X., & Yu, G. (2021). Exploring the online behavior of users of online depression-focused communities: Comparing communities with different management types. *Psychology Research and Behavior Management*, 1707–1724.

Weiss, R. (2020). Menopause cafés: It's good to talk. *Maturitas, 132*, 79–80.

Wilson, S., Mogan, S., Coulson, N., & Tham, J. S. (2022). Exploring the role of a WhatsApp online community in supporting the needs of women living with endometriosis in Malaysia: An interview study. *Asian Women, 38*(1), 59–76.

Wright, W. J., Howdle, C., Coulson, N. S., & De Simoni, A. (2024). Exploring the types of social support exchanged by survivors of pediatric stroke and their families in an online peer support community: Qualitative thematic analysis. *Journal of Medical Internet Research, 26*, e49440.

Yadav, D., Dabas, K., Malik, P., Bhandari, A., & Singh, P. (2022, April). "Should I visit the clinic": Analyzing Whatsapp-mediated online health support for expectant and new mothers in rural India. *Proceedings of the 2022 CHI Conference on Human Factors in Computing Systems* (pp. 1–20).

Yazdkhasti, M., Keshavarz, M., Khoei, E. M., Hosseini, A., Esmaeilzadeh, S., Pebdani, M. A., & Jafarzadeh, H. (2012). The effect of support group method on quality of life in post-menopausal women. *Iranian Journal of Public Health, 41*, 78–84.

Yeshua-Katz, D. (2021). The role of communication affordances in post-traumatic stress disorder Facebook and WhatsApp support groups. *International Journal of Environmental Research and Public Health, 18*, Article 4576.
Ziebland, S., & Wyke, S. (2012). Health and illness in a connected world: How might sharing experiences on the internet affect people's health? *The Milbank Quarterly, 90*(2), 219–249.

7

Conclusions and Future Directions

Abstract This chapter seeks to review the findings from the preceding chapters and to draw together the key take-home points. We will use this chapter to evaluate how the different digital health technologies examined in the book play a role in health communication around menopause and how they contribute to the current debates around medicalisation and empowerment. In addition, the chapter reflects on the current gaps in the literature and identifies potential limitations with the current research base including sampling and inclusivity. We highlight areas that remain underexplored in relation to digital health technologies and menopause then conclude with suggestions for future research alongside practical implications for increasing access to information and support for individuals going through menopause.

Keywords Digital health technologies · Medicalisation · Patient empowerment · Epistemic injustice · Representation · Artificial intelligence

E. Sillence and A. Osborne, *Digital Health Technologies and the Menopause*, Palgrave Studies in Cyberpsychology, https://doi.org/10.1007/978-3-032-25909-7_7

7.1 Summary of Findings

Throughout the book, we have sought to illustrate how different digital health technologies play a role in menopause information and support. The different DHTs support seeking, accessing, and consuming information. Whilst some DHTs have provided an information resource for over 20 years, others such as podcasts and menopause apps are relatively newcomers to the space. These DHTs have allowed women to track their own personal health data and provided an alternative way of accessing and consuming information and support, in more private yet more accessible ways. We have seen how the type of menopause information content has changed and adapted and how the key voices and providers have expanded and diversified.

We begin this final chapter with a quick recap of each of the preceding chapters. We then delve into the key take-home messages before considering implications and future research directions.

Chapter 2 highlighted a plethora of websites on menopause. There is a lot of overlap in terms of content, and unless information seekers have a specific question in mind, it can feel overwhelming. Our studies showed there was a reliance on the NHS as a starting point, although the landscape of information providers is diverse, with a lot of private healthcare providers, media, and retail organisations offering menopause information and support.

Chapter 3 showed that menopause apps are viewed positively by women particularly as a way of tracking and visualising their personal health data. Apps vary in terms of their features and usability, but better-quality apps allow content to be tailored and provide users with access to data visualisations, information, and community features. Apps were seen as a useful way of improving communication with HCPs.

In Chapter 4, we examined menopause podcasts noting from our studies and others that the format whilst underexplored is engaging for women seeking information on menopause. The accessibility of the podcasts, their private nature, and their authentic and intimate style make them a popular way for gleaning more specific information as well as for providing the reassurance of 'not being alone'.

Chapter 5 shone a light on social media and menopause influencers. Whilst most of our participants used social media, only a few were actively engaged with social media for menopause information. The narrative of social media posts can be quite polarising, and women preferred less overtly negative or positive messages, whilst a larger scale survey study found that negative framing of menopause narratives increased negative affect around menopause, with women feeling more anxious and more worried about menopause.

Chapter 6 considered peer support for people going through menopause. Peers continue to provide an important source of information and support for women, and digital technology allows access to a wider range of peer experiences. The tone of the online community and the design of the platform can affect how comfortable women feel about sharing their experiences and engaging with the support.

Across the chapters more broadly, we see that women find DHTs a valuable resource in accessing and consuming information and support on menopause. They find the information useful and take comfort in the knowledge that others are encountering similar experiences. Women want to know more about menopause and often feel poorly educated through traditional routes. Women use the DHTs to listen to other people's accounts, to validate their own experiences, to find tips and advice, to find answers to specific issues, to reflect on symptoms, and to log and track their own health data.

The value of the DHTs depends, however, on where a woman is within her menopause journey, the symptoms she is experiencing, and the treatments she is taking or has tried. It also depends on the extent to which she is supported by friends, family, work colleagues, and importantly her HCP. Whilst all women were familiar with websites, mobile apps and podcasts also provided women with access to information and support. In fact, the different DHTs offered distinct affordances, affective factors, and agency (Lupton & Maslen, 2019), although there were also similarities. The ways in which participants engaged with these technologies were further shaped by their familiarity with the technology and their personal preferences for format, tone, and style around digital health information.

Importantly, DHTs only play a part of the picture, with most women still valuing in-place support and information coming via HCPs. They value the tailored approach and prefer a more holistic approach to women's health and wellbeing being taken. This suggests that the role of DHTs is not to replace but to support traditional forms of menopause information and support.

7.2 The Framing of Menopause

Across the chapters, we have seen evidence of the different ways in which menopause is framed from being a natural, biological event to a distressing, debilitating process. This was particularly apparent in Chapters 2 and 5 in which participants commented on the contradictory narratives, the varied experiences, and the extreme representations. These differing framings are perhaps to be expected given the uniqueness of the menopause experience. In fact, as Cahn et al. (2022) put it, menopause can be a women's health issue that is both 'exceptionalised' and 'unexceptional' (p. 79), and this is a problem for health communication. These different narratives can impact upon how women feel about menopause. Whilst Davina McCall's programmes (Channel 4, 2021) and other menopause influencers have raised the profile of menopause, which is undoubtedly a positive thing, it has tended to come with a strong focus on a negative and or very medicalised framing. These framings highlight the potential debilitating symptoms which can make women feel anxious about the menopause in general. Work in our research group shows that different social media narratives can impact affective responses to menopause, so that distress narratives which focus heavily on hormone deficiency and difficult experiences can lead to increased anxiety, worry, and confusion. This resonates with recent work that found that participants judge memorable peri/menopause messages as negative or ambivalent, suggesting cognitive biases favouring negative menopause information (Rubinsky et al., 2025). A diverse expression of menopause narratives online would better reflect the highly individual nature of the transition, resonate with more women's lived experiences, and help reduce stigma and open discussion (de Salis et al.,

2018; Orgad & Rottenberg, 2024). Across our studies, many of our participants rejected a one-size-fits-all or overly medicalised narrative of menopause, highlighting the need for resources to be inclusive, capturing a broader representation of menopause experiences, perspectives, and treatment options.

7.3 Representation in Menopause Information

A common limitation of DHTs for menopause concerns representation. Feeling represented by DHTs is an important factor in determining their use, and many women feel that their experience is not represented online or digitally (Lopez Burst et al. 2024). Our participants did not always know how to label themselves in relation to menopause or did not relate to images of grey-haired women under the banner post-menopausal, making it difficult to find a representative experience on the DHTs. More broadly, there is recognition that menopause experiences in the media often foreground white, middle-class, cis gender accounts (Jermyn, 2025). Menopause information is often lacking for specific groups, including neurodiverse women (Grant et al., 2025) and those in medically induced or surgical menopause (Funnell et al., 2025).

Despite the recognition of the need for greater diversity of menopausal experiences, a great deal of the literature still relates to high-income countries with less attention to underserved communities (Shams et al., 2025). Researchers, including ourselves, need to ensure that a greater range of voices are included (Drysdale et al., 2025), diversifying our participant population and capturing a more accurate account of women's experiences. We also need to ensure that women themselves are involved in the development of appropriate and relevant digital resources. Biases or poor representation in the research literature may be mirrored in the algorithms powering FemTech. In menstrual tracking apps, for example, there are concerns that the diversity of menstrual experiences is diminished through homogenised algorithms and predictions (Hammond & Burdon, 2024). Finally, it is important to acknowledge that not everyone has access to DHTs for menopause. Digital exclusion remains a problem for many, and access to services for menopause more broadly is often geographically diverse.

7.4 Empowerment and Epistemic Injustice: Individual Responsibility

In Chapter 3, women described some of the difficulties they had experienced in seeking information and support on menopause from their HCPs. They discussed not being believed or taken seriously, fuelling a sense of epistemic injustice in which women's own knowledge about their bodies is not believed (Fricker, 2007). Women went on to describe their use of menopause apps as 'empowering' increasing their knowledge on menopause and their sense of control over the process. It could be argued that the increased focus on menopause from different groups including celebrities, influencers, and the media more broadly may also impact expectations for individuals to 'manage' their own menopause through a range of promoted solutions and practices (Corus et al., 2025). However, this highlights a tension in which menopause narratives highlight the systemic and structural ways in which women are failed through menopause, including poor access to menopause clinics and gendered inequalities in care, yet offer solutions that focus on personal endeavour (Orgad & Rottenberg, 2024). Whilst menopause can be an intensely personal issue, the current narrative to some extent puts the burden of responsibility on the individual, forgetting that menopause impacts more broadly and that societal and system shifts are required (see Thomas et al., 2024 for further discussion). This tension resonates with the literature on patient empowerment more broadly which is often defined in individual terms with research failing to adequately address the impactful structural barriers or systemic issues (Agner & Braun, 2018). Martha Hickey, lead author of a recent Lancet menopause series, has advocated for a "move beyond describing and treating symptoms to a broader model of empowering women to manage this life transition" (Samarasekera, 2024 p. 1). This approach to empowerment argues for access to information and tools to aid decision-making alongside access to supportive and informed clinicians and considers broader aspects of women's lives including the workplace environment and broader societal issues around stigma and gender-based ageism (Hickey et al., 2024).

7.5 What Next for Digital Health Technologies?

There was variability in terms of the information covered across the different DHTs, and this points to gaps in information provision that could and should be filled by DHTs going forward. Across all the DHTs, there was a focus on peri/menopausal symptoms and understanding the basics of menopause, treatment options, and lifestyle changes that can help to alleviate symptoms. Other topics received less widespread coverage, for example, there was patchy content on menopause and the workplace. The top three websites in Chapter 2 varied in relation to this topic. It was briefly mentioned on the NHS website, whilst it constituted a main tab on the homepage of Balance. There is a research literature looking at menopause in the workplace. Studies have reported on women's accounts of how they would like to be treated by their managers and employers during menopause and their preferences for conversations with line managers about menopause (Hardy et al., 2017, 2018). Cronin et al. (2023) found that nurses would value DHTs that support connection, information, and tracking and called for more evidence-based women-centred information to support women going through menopause in the workplace.

An online organisational toolkit has recently been trialled across eight UK-based organisations with promising results on multiple measures, including menopause awareness, problematic hot flush frequency, job performance, and work ability (Hardy et al., 2025). These toolkits emphasise the importance of a whole organisation approach—managers, colleagues, friends, and family. Access to information and support via organisations may be one way of reducing the burden on individuals to search through multiple sources, although, as Orgad and Rottenberg (2024) note, menopause support in the workplace is heavily dependent on the nature of the work and the workplace.

Information on sex and relationships during menopause was also covered less comprehensively on the DHTs than other topics. We know that women often report sexual difficulties during menopause including reduced interest in sexual activity and vaginal dryness and can find it difficult to discuss these issues with HCPs or friends and family (Bulut et al., 2025). Menopause may play a role in relationship difficulties (Caico, 2011) and whilst wider changes in a woman's mid-life context may also be important here (Dillaway, 2007, 2008, 2020), some women directly attribute relationship difficulties as arising from peri/menopause (Hayfield et al., 2024). Lack of knowledge about menopause can impact the ability to cope with relationship difficulties, whilst we know that general menopause education reduces sexual symptoms such as changes in sexual desire, avoiding intimacy, or vaginal dryness during intercourse in menopausal women (Keye et al., 2023). There is still scope for DHTs to provide more detailed and targeted information and support for women in this context. Information on websites was once again mixed (see Chapter 2), and it may be that certain DHTs, for example podcasts, lend themselves to more discreet information and support.

7.5.1 The Role of AI in Menopause Information and Support

As with other health topics, the role of AI has been increasing rapidly in recent years.

Women may benefit from data from wearable devices alerting users to symptom triggers (Ang & Hillard, 2025), and AI chatbots could provide personalised information and support for women going through menopause. We already know that in related fields such as pregnancy and early parenthood, parents appreciate the information and emotional support offered by chatbots (Chua et al., 2023), and in a small-scale review of AI for endometriosis (Oliveira et al., 2024), AI responses were scored as accurate. There is also an emerging literature base on trust in AI and health information, with a notable proportion of the population now using Large Language Models (LLMs), e.g. ChatGPT for health information (Yun & Bickmore, 2025). Findings regarding trust are mixed with some studies suggesting that AI is trusted more than Google for health information searches at least in experimental settings (Sun et al., 2024) whilst other studies have found little difference in terms of perceived quality and trustworthiness across sources (search engines, health websites, apps, and AI) although people were less likely to adhere to AI information (Yun & Bickmore, 2025). Understanding how AI will be further integrated into DHTs for menopause is an ongoing line of research.

7.6 Summary and Final Thoughts

Throughout our studies, it remains clear that despite the perceived and the experienced difficulties with accessing medical information and support, women would in many cases still view their HCP as their first port of call regarding menopause. This would suggest a need for improved training for HCPs, especially GPs in the UK, around menopause. GPs do not feel they have enough support to be able to advise and treat women with menopausal symptoms appropriately and menopause training needs to be improved in medical school and in GP training (Dintakurti et al., 2022). Of course, this is not straightforward and must be viewed within the context of an under-resourced and time-constrained NHS.

The role of digital resources is therefore perhaps best envisaged as one that supplements but does not replace traditional information and support. Thinking of improved touchpoints for women to engage with HCPs about menopause could facilitate more productive integration of digital resources such as menopause apps into conversations with HCPs. Our participants suggested combining menopause sessions with women's health checks at 40 (an initiative that has recently been announced in the UK, (Department of Health and Social Care, 2025)), or at cervical screening appointments. It is clear that there is a need for a more sustained approach to menopause education throughout the lifespan (Harper et al., 2024).

Going forward, the developers of DHTs need to consider how they become more inclusive, how they represent women at different stages of their menopause journey, and how they use accessible language to allow women to engage with a more varied and balanced set of menopause narratives that avoid demonising the experience but also avoid oversimplifying or trivialising the issues for many—no small task!

Many women get their information and support about menstrual health from within their families in particular from their mother. Whilst this is not always possible, the desire for intergenerational information is strong (Field-Springer et al., 2018). With that in mind, we end this chapter and the book with an example of menopause legacies, a project focused on capturing experiences of menopause that can be both useful to women experiencing menopause, but importantly can serve as an important source of information and support for future generations. Chopra et al. (2024) asked women to capture information about their menopause and to think about what would be important to pass on to future generations. Women wanted to share their experiences and advise their children on how to prepare and make sense of menopause. For some women, it was important to capture this menopause experience separately—whilst others embedded it within a broader lifelogging context. Women expressed preferences for using digital and non-digital ways of sharing including paper-based journals and voice notes. Importantly, women wanted to be able to share these intergenerational resources in person—again the importance of integrating the digital with in-person resources. DHTs remain an important part of the toolkit but women still want and value in-place, personal contact, and support as they navigate through menopause.

References

Agner, J., & Braun, K. L. (2018). Patient empowerment: A critique of individualism and systematic review of patient perspectives. *Patient Education and Counseling, 101*(12), 2054–2064.

Ang, S. B., & Hillard, T. (2025). Preparing for the future: Artificial intelligence in menopausal health care. *Climacteric, 28*(2), 95–97.

Bulut, H., Hinchliff, S., Ali, P., & Piercy, H. (2025). Women's experiences of intimate and sexual relationships during menopause: A qualitative synthesis. *Journal of Clinical Nursing, 34*(5), 1543–1554.

Cahn, N. R., Crawford, B. J., & Waldman, E. G. (2022). *Managing and monitoring the menopausal body* (p. 41). University of Chicago Legal Forum.

Caico, C. (2011). Do perimenopausal and menopausal symptoms affect the marital relationship? *Journal of Research in Nursing, 18*(3), 204–215.

Channel 4. (2021). *Davina McCall: Sex, myths and the menopause*. https://www.channel4.com/programmes/davina-mccall-sex-myths-and-the-menopause

Chopra, S., Orii, L., Juarez, K., Tieanklin, N., Fogarty, J., & Munson, S. A. (2024). Menopause legacies: Designing to record and share experiences of menopause across generations. *Proceedings of the ACM on Human-Computer Interaction, 8*(CSCW2), 1–37.

Chua, J. Y. X., Choolani, M., Chee, C. Y. I., Chan, Y. H., Lalor, J. G., Chong, Y. S., & Shorey, S. (2023). Insights of parents and parents-to-be in using chatbots to improve their preconception, pregnancy, and postpartum health: A mixed studies review. *Journal of Midwifery & Women's Health, 68*(4), 480–489.

Corus, C., Saatcioglu, B., & Sandikci, O. (2025). Gendered consumer responsibilization: The constitution of menopausal women as responsible feminine consumer subjects. *Journal of Consumer Research, 52*(2), 351–371.

Cronin, C., Bidwell, G., Carey, J., Donevant, S., Hughes, K. A., Kaunonen, M., Mather, C., & Wilson, R. (2023). Exploring digital interventions to facilitate coping and discomfort for nurses experiencing the menopause in the workplace: An international qualitative study. *Journal of Advanced Nursing, 79*(10), 3760–3775.

de Salis, I., Owen-Smith, A., Donovan, J. L., & Lawlor, D. A. (2018). Experiencing menopause in the UK: The interrelated narratives of normality, distress, and transformation. *Journal of Women & Aging, 30*(6), 520–540.

Department of Health and Social Care (2025). *Major NHS update brings menopause into routine health checks*. https://www.gov.uk/government/news/major-nhs-update-brings-menopause-into-routine-health-checks. Accessed 7.11.25.

Dillaway, H. (2020). Living in uncertain times: Experiences of menopause and reproductive aging. In *The Palgrave handbook of critical menstruation studies* (pp. 253–268).

Dillaway, H. E. (2007). "Am I similar to my mother?" how women make sense of menopause using family background. *Women & Health, 46*(1), 79–97.

Dillaway, H. E. (2008). "Why can't you control this?" how women's interactions with intimate partners define menopause and family. *Journal of Women & Aging, 20*(1–2), 47–64.

Dintakurti, N., Kalyanasundaram, S., Jha, P., & Talaulikar, V. (2022). An online survey and interview of GPs in the UK for assessing their satisfaction regarding the medical training curriculum and NICE guidelines for the management of menopause. *Post Reproductive Health, 28*(3), 137–141.

Drysdale, K., Burton-Clark, I., & Moline, K. (2025). Reimagining menopause by expanding assumptions shaping research: A scoping review of gender and sexuality diverse people's experiences and expectations. *International Journal of Transgender Health*, 1–16.

Field-Springer, K., Randall-Griffiths, D., & Reece, C. (2018). From menarche to menopause: Understanding multigenerational reproductive health milestones. *Health Communication, 33*(6), 733–742.

Fricker, M. (2007). *Epistemic injustice: Power and the ethics of knowing*. Oxford University Press.

Funnell, E. L., McConnell, F., Martin-Key, N. A., Qian, L., Babbitt, K., & Bahn, S. (2025). Understanding experiences of and unmet needs in online searches for menopause information: An exploratory survey. *JMIR Formative Research, 9*, e75335.

Grant, A., Axbey, H., Holloway, W., Caemawr, S., Craine, M., Lim, H., McKenzie, K., & Ellis, R. (2025). *Autism and the menopause transition: A mixed-methods systematic review*. Autism in Adulthood.

Hammond, E., & Burdon, M. (2024). Intimate harms and menstrual cycle tracking apps. *Computer Law and Security Review, 55*.

Hardy, C., Clarry, L., Hunter, M. S., & Griffiths, A. (2025). Assessing the effects of an online organisational toolkit to support menopause in the workplace (MENO-kit). *Maturitas, 199*, 108304.

Hardy, C., Griffiths, A., & Hunter, M. S. (2017). What do working menopausal women want? A qualitative investigation into women's perspectives on employer and line manager support. *Maturitas, 101*, 37–41.

Hardy, C., Thorne, E., Griffiths, A., & Hunter, M. (2018). Tackling the taboo: Talking menopause-related problems at work. *International Journal of Workplace Health Management, 12*(1), 28–38.

Harper, J., Keay, N., Rowe, F., Alstyne, P. V., & Tariq, S. (2024). The time has come for a UK-wide menopause education and support programme: InTune. *Women's Health, 20*, 17455057241277535.

Hayfield, N., Moore, H., & Terry, G. (2024). "Friends? Supported. Partner? Not so much...": Women's experiences of friendships, family, and relationships during perimenopause and menopause. *Feminism & Psychology, 34*(3), 443–463.

Hickey, M., LaCroix, A. Z., Doust, J., Mishra, G. D., & Ussher, J. (2024). An empowerment model for managing menopause. *The Lancet, 403*, 947–957.

Jermyn, D. (2025). Whose menopause revolution? Investigating the UK'S 'Davina effect' and the contemporary menopause market. *European Journal of Cultural Studies, 28*(4), 1039–1057.

Keye, C., Varley, J., & Patton, D. (2023). The impact of menopause education on quality of life among menopausal women: A systematic review with meta-analysis. *Climacteric, 26*(5), 419–427.

Lopez Burst, E., Ciolfi Felice, M., & O'Kane, A. A. (2024, May). Using and appropriating technology to support the menopause journey in the UK. *Proceedings.*

Lupton, D., & Maslen, S. (2019). How women use digital technologies for health: Qualitative interview and focus group study. *Journal of Medical Internet Research, 21*(1), e11481.

Oliveira, J. A., Eskandar, K., Kar, E., de Oliveira, F. R., & Filho, A. L. D. S. (2024). Understanding AI'S role in endometriosis patient education and evaluating its information and accuracy: Systematic review. *JMIR AI, 3*, e64593.

Orgad, S., & Rottenberg, C. (2024). The menopause moment: The rising visibility of 'the change' in UK news coverage. *European Journal of Cultural Studies, 27*(4), 519–539.

Rubinsky, V., Tolman, C., & Cooke-Jackson, A. (2025). "Just deal with it": Memorable messages about menopause as anticipatory education. *American Journal of Sexuality Education*, 1–26.

Samarasekera, U. (2024). Martha Hickey: Responding to the complexity of menopause. *The Lancet, 403*(10430), 893.

Shams, A., Aurangzaib, Z., & Sherazi, S. F. A. (2025). Breaking the silence: Understanding menopause, stigma, and support in under served communities. *Journal of Medical & Health Sciences Review, 2*(2).

Sun, X., Ma, R., Zhao, X., Li, Z., Lindqvist, J., Ali, A. E., & Bosch, J. A. (2024). Trusting the search: Unraveling human trust in health information from Google and ChatGPT. *arXiv preprint* https://arxiv.org/abs/2403.09987.

Thomas, S. L., Randle, M., & White, S. L. (2024). (re)framing menopause: A comprehensive public health approach. *Health Promotion International, 39*(3), Article daae052.
Yun, H. S., & Bickmore, T. (2025). Online health information–seeking in the era of large language models: Cross-sectional web-based survey study. *Journal of Medical Internet Research, 27*, Article e68560.

Index

E. Sillence and A. Osborne, *Digital Health Technologies and the Menopause*, Palgrave Studies in Cyberpsychology, https://doi.org/10.1007/978-3-032-25909-7

The manufacturer's authorised representative in the EU is Springer Nature Customer Service Centre GmbH, Europaplatz 3, 69115 Heidelberg, Germany. If you have any concerns regarding our products, please contact ProductSafety@springernature.com

Printed and bound by CPI Group (UK) Ltd, Croydon, CR0 4YY
16/09/2026
02217792-0001